PRAISE FOR *WITHIN*

"*Habib Sadeghi is an insightful, kind man who approaches healing in a fresh and uncomplicated way. If one is able to acknowledge that illness is created by an imbalance in the body, and that one's state of mind and emotional well-being are integral to the overall health of the body, then Habib has practical suggestions on how to achieve a new realm of health and healing.*"

—**Tim Robbins**, actor, director, producer

"*Dr. Sadeghi has shown me how my outside often reflects my inside; how our minds and bodies mirror each other. He has helped me a great deal, and I hope that through this book more people can enjoy the benefit of his compassion.*"

—**Chris Martin**, singer/songwriter, Coldplay

"*When you locate a person in your world that is able to understand who you are at a very deep level — you rejoice at your great good fortune. When you locate a doctor in your world who is able to know what is going on throughout your body in a holistic way — you also rejoice at such a fortunate discovery. When you find that the doctor you have met is also such an intuitive person — you are permitted to spend a few moments in completely honest disbelief . . . it is totally natural. Dr. Habib Sadeghi is such a person and such a doctor . . . welcome to the wonderful world of life's realizations and health filled resolutions that reach way beyond your brightest expectations.*"

—**Guru Singh, D.D. m.s.s.,** spiritual teacher/author

"*I don't think I've come across anyone who understands more about the mind/body connection when it comes to changing our health or our lives than Dr. Sadeghi. In fact, he's living proof of it.*"

—**Emily Blunt**, actor

"*Dr. Sadeghi approaches overwhelming issues with a soft and gentle approach. He gives us support to life's challenges in a way that removes fear and shame. We have the power to change our lives and Dr. Sadeghi helps you to help yourself.*"

—**Stella McCartney**, fashion designer

"At last, the time has come where sound medical practice includes the well-being of the patient and not merely the alleviation of his or her symptoms. And I am not aware of anyone who is more at the forefront of this initiative than Habib Sadeghi. I personally know him well and am certain that he is one of the few who venture the possibility that Love and weight release are directly related— much less how to utilize this information in service to health. Thank you Habib."

—**H. Ronald Hulnick**, Ph.D., President, University of Santa Monica and co-author of *Loyalty to Your Soul: The Heart of Spiritual Psychology*

"Dr. Sadeghi reminds us that the key to unlock the door of healing has always been right in our hands. His heartfelt words and lessons guide us to the place where what we've been searching for all along has been hiding in plain sight, Within."

—**Sara Bordo**, film producer and author of *Woman Rising*

"Dr. Habib Sadeghi presents a gentle yet deeply powerful methodology for understanding the impact our emotions and thoughts have on our bodies. He puts healing within reach of those who struggle with weight issues and anyone else on the journey of seeking a more fulfilling life experience. WiTHIN is a clarion to stop, look, and listen to our authentic selves by providing us with achievable strategies to overcome past traumas which may negatively impact our health and happiness. Through bravely sharing his own personal healing journey, Dr. Sadeghi's wisdom, warmth and acceptance reach through the pages in a reassuring yet straight-shooting approach that motivates and inspires."

—**Mary Gordon**, founder of Roots of Empathy

"I'm writing this from a 6-month sabbatical in Italy, wearing my 'skinny' clothes! That's something I could never have done had I not learned the simple but powerful secret of self-love from Dr. Sadeghi. His empowering approach is a revelation that will open your eyes to the fact that you are not broken. You are whole right now. Nothing needs to be 'fixed'. You just need to remember who you really are and Dr. Sadeghi gives you the road map to rise to your own magnificence."

—**Renee Croce,** fundraising consultant

"Dr. Sadeghi clearly captures the multidimensional levels of weight-related health issues in Within. His life experience in medicine, teaching, and his own healing journey from cancer back to perfect health illuminates a path for others to follow. His expertise and understanding provide real solutions for problems that affect millions."

—**Alesandra Rain**, author and prescription drug expert

"Dr. Sadeghi possesses an unquenchable thirst for knowledge and every page of Within overflows with the depth of his experience. It's a rare and savory gift that goes well beyond why we eat and explores the deeper questions of why we're on the planet. If you're hungry for a terrific book, better health or a better life, I can't recommend Within highly enough."

—**Richard Martini**, author of *Flipside: A Tourist's Guide on How to Navigate the Afterlife*

"Dr. Sadeghi reaches through the pages and speaks to your soul in the only way a person can who has 'been there'. The depth of his compassion and power of his personal journey will redefine everything you ever thought was possible."

—**Katherine Woodward Thomas**, author of *Calling in "The One": 7 Weeks to Attract the Love of Your Life*

"No one on Earth understands the heart/mind/body connection better than Dr. Sadeghi. I know from my own personal experience that where others fail to make a difference in your heath, Dr. Sadeghi succeeds. He is a truly a life changer."

—**Brad Falchuk**, co-creator and executive producer of *Glee* and *American Horror Story*

"Dr. Sadeghi's influence on my life has far exceeded physical healing. He has elevated my consciousness, awareness and understanding of what it means to be a responsible citizen of the planet. In a rapidly changing world, his sound and practical wisdom is a godsend."

—**Matt Bohmer**, actor

"Dr. Sadeghi is more than a physician. He is a modern day alchemist. He has empowered my entire family on a path to wellness through his integrative and conscious practice. As a result, he has not only improved our health; he has improved our lives."

—**Stacy Sher**, film producer

"From 'Wait Loss' to Weight loss, Dr. Sadeghi identifies and heals the obstacles that are keeping you from the health accomplishments you desire. YOU can become the star performer in an amazing life as Dr. Sadeghi provides the tools to activate change on many levels. You'll be able to choose and accomplish goals you never thought possible and celebrate every step."

—**Tracy Anderson**, personal trainer, fitness expert, and author

WITHIN

A Spiritual Awakening to Love & Weight Loss

Dr. Habib Sadeghi
Co-founder, BeHive of Healing, Center for Integrative Medicine

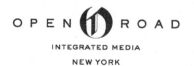

OPEN ROAD
INTEGRATED MEDIA
NEW YORK

Figures on pages 22, 34, 36, 40, 63, 64, 112, 115, 136, and 162 credited to Susie Liptak

978-1-4976-6115-8

This edition published in 2014 by Open Road Integrated Media, Inc.
345 Hudson Street
New York, NY 10014
www.openroadmedia.com

CONTENTS

Dedication...III

Acknowledgments..IV

Foreword... VII

Introduction..1

Chapter 1: The Real You 8

Chapter 2: Believe It or Not 19

Chapter 3: Feel It to Heal It..41

Chapter 4: What Did You Say? - *The Power of Words*.................. 50

Chapter 5: Consciousness is King.................................. 60

Chapter 6: Goodbye to You - *Letting Go of Your Story* 73

Chapter 7: A Life in Pictures - *The Power of Visualization* 82

Chapter 8: Myth & Madness - *Beauty Myths & Surgery Madness*.............. 90

Chapter 9: How do I look in these genes? - *The Revolution of Epigenetics*........ 110

Chapter 10: The Pleasure Principle - *The Selflessness of Selfishness* 121

Chapter 11: Head Space - *The Miracle of Meditation* 131

Chapter 12: The Rhythm of Life - *Expansion & Contraction* 144

Chapter 13: The Pillars of Personal Change 157

    I Self-Love 157

    II Self-Acceptance.. 165

    III Self-Forgiveness.. 169

Chapter 14: My Story 181

Chapter 15: Your Larger Destiny 192

Chapter 16: A Final Word 199

The Program 201

About the Healing Institute of Beings (HIB)...................... 268

To:

My beloved God
Whose love feeds my soul daily

Dr. Shahrzad (Sherry) Sami
Meeting you, my beloved soulmate, for the first time
in front of Columbia University transformed my consciousness
and made me the best version of myself.

Hafez Sami Sadeghi
Our son. My poet and prophet that taught me courage and playfulness.

Hannah Sami Sadeghi
Our daughter. The gift from God that made me
a believer in the unseen world of angels.

My parents
Who proved that encouragement, perseverance and unconditional love
is the only way to bring the best out of a child. I'm living proof of it.

Dr. Mehrdad Sadeghi
My brother. The world renowned cardiologist whose embodiment of
patience and humility taught me the essence of these virtues.

Dr. Mehran Sadeghi
My brother. Although he's a lawyer by day,
I believe he's really a wizard in disguise.

ACKNOWLEDGMENTS

I would like to acknowledge those whose ceaseless dedication, companionship and guidance make my life a richer experience just by having the privilege of knowing and working with them. Thank you for being a part of my journey. I love you all.

Sri Madhuji
Your patience and passion to change the world inspires me daily.

Be Hive of Healing Team
You have proven that miracles ARE a natural daily occurrence.

Dr. Gary H. Mason
Your support is invaluable. I'm proud to call you my colleague and partner.

Luke Cowles
Your guidance helped me find my voice
and gave me the courage to share it with the world.

Dr. Ron & Mary Hulnick
My spiritual parents who whispered "HU",
the address to God's heart, while soul gazing.

Stevollah Forbes Hardison
You taught me to keep Mother Death close by agreeing to read your eulogy.

Byron Katie
You're one of my favorite dancing partners!
Thank you for teaching me to dare to be homeless, and ASK!

Kamran Golestaneh
My climbing partner and confidant. For 26 years, your friendship has been a safety net of loving that has rescued me more times than I can count.

My Life Coaches
That's you, all my patients, teachers, colleagues and friends whose love, knowledge and guidance have brought me through the last 43 years to the place I am today . . . the world of awareness and gratitude.

"Last night as I was sleeping,
I dreamt—marvelous error!—
that a spring was breaking
out in my heart.
I said: Along which secret aqueduct,
Oh water, are you coming to me,
water of a new life
that I have never drunk?
Last night as I was sleeping,
I dreamt—marvelous error!—
that I had a beehive
here inside my heart.
And the golden bees
were making white combs
and sweet honey
from my old failures.
Last night as I was sleeping,
I dreamt—marvelous error!—
that a fiery sun was giving
light inside my heart.
It was fiery because I felt
warmth as from a hearth,
and sun because it gave light
and brought tears to my eyes.
Last night as I slept,
I dreamt—marvelous error!—
that it was God I had
here inside my heart. "

—Antonio Machado

All proceeds from *WITHIN* go to benefit:

Roots of Empathy
www.rootsofempathy.org

University of Santa Monica
www.universityofsantamonica.edu

&

Healing Institute of Beings
www.healingbeings.org

FOREWORD

〰

When you get to a certain point in life, you begin to realize there are larger forces at work in the universe, or at least you suspect there might be. Maybe things don't happen randomly. Maybe everything does have a purpose. Maybe my role in this life isn't what it appears to be, and just maybe, I'm more powerful than I ever allowed myself to believe. Then, you meet someone who's living from this awareness, and it changes everything.

That's how I felt when I met Dr. Habib Sadeghi. His expertise in integrative medicine is what brings patients to him from all over the world, but it's really his understanding of how the mind, body, and spirit are connected that creates dramatic changes in people's lives, mine included. He understands what much of modern medicine is only now beginning to explore. Our thoughts and emotions have far more influence on our health than we've ever imagined. In fact, it's so significant that you might think of our bodies as just the physical printouts of what's already going on in our hearts. Dr. Sadeghi knows that, regardless of the challenges someone might be facing, healing has to start at a deeper level for it to be complete and lasting.

Since 2008, I've been a part of the Stand Up to Cancer (SU2C) organization that raises funding for cancer research. Every other year, the program holds a telethon to raise money for grant awards that will go to emerging research projects around the world. Celebrities, musicians, professional athletes, and world-renowned cancer researchers take part in the event to bring awareness to the issue and provide updates on finding a cure. Last year, we raised $81 million, for a total of $137 million since the SU2C movement began.

In 2012, I wanted to bring a new perspective to the SU2C event. I wanted to give a voice to the emerging science of how the mind and body communicate with each other in working to produce our state of health. For me, that voice is Dr. Sadeghi. He knows more about the mind/body balance than anyone I know. It's not just because he's an international expert on integrative medicine. It's because he has the kind of experience that can't be taught. He's a doctor who's also been a patient. He's been to the edge of what looked like an insurmountable situation and overcome it. He didn't just survive. He thrives by applying the life principles you'll read in this book. Yes, he really does practice what he preaches.

I truly believe that the best teacher anyone can have is someone who's "been there" and Dr. Sadeghi has been there . . . and back. That's why last year he became one of the first osteopathic physicians to ever participate in SU2C, providing his life-changing wisdom alongside researchers and Nobel Laureates from around the world.

I like to think of Dr. Sadeghi's approach to healing as active compassion. He has a way of intuitively connecting with people that makes them feel instantly understood, safe, and at ease. He also gives them the tools they need to affect real change in their lives. That's more than just encouraging. It's empowering. Isn't that what we all want during the times we feel vulnerable? We want our power back.

It's my privilege to call Dr. Sadeghi my friend. He's brought clarity to my life in ways that only someone with an old soul truly can. I guess that's why some people actually do call him the Old Soul Doctor. As you read these pages, I've no doubt that his insights will touch you in very much the same way. While the focus of Within might be on weight loss, please remember that the principles it teaches can be applied to any challenge you're facing. Whether you want to lose weight, improve your health, repair your relationships, or something else, the cause of how we're creating our personal world is always found Within. That's where you'll find the answer, too.

Gwyneth Paltrow
Los Angeles
2013

I, Lord went wandering like a strayed sheep,
seeking Thee with anxious reasoning without,
whilst Thou was within me.
I went round the streets and squares of the city seeking Thee,
and I found Thee not, because in vain
*I sought without for him who was **within** myself.*

—*St. Augustine*

INTRODUCTION
WE'RE ALL HUNGRY

Everyone seems to be sprinting through life, driven by their cravings for success, companionship, money, romance, fame, or some other unsettled desire. It's the next relationship, higher paying job, big house, or perfect body that will *finally* satiate us and give us a sense of worthiness to simply exist in the world. It has to. That's why we keep running.

The truth is we're all searching. What we're really looking for is a sense of direction when our personal world seems out of control—a *knowingness* that assures us that we have a purpose in this world and that we're *safe* in it as we struggle to find that path. Eventually, most of us come to realize this "blessed assurance" that grounds and guides our lives through the tough times does not come from external experiences or expensive possessions. If it did, we'd never read another headline about some millionaire who seemed to "have it all" who jumped out of an office window when the stock market took a plunge, or a beautiful movie star who's returned to rehab.

Knowing what doesn't fill that inner void is progress. It's half the battle. Finding what *does* work—that missing "peace" is another challenge altogether. Until we find it, we'll continue to run. Running, however, implies that we're actually getting somewhere. We're not. We're a culture on a treadmill, continually pursuing the same things we know don't offer the happiness we desperately

I

desire. Even lab rats, when shocked several times in a maze, will take another route. As human beings, we can spend our entire lives retreading the same road. Our bad habits, negative emotions, and erroneous beliefs are driving forces that keep us banging into a wall like a windup toy that's run out of floor space. It's time to turn around and take a completely different direction. After all, it was American author Mark Twain who said, "If you do what you've always done, you'll get what you've always gotten."

So how do we get off the treadmill? What's the answer for a culture that's more than just hungry? It's starving to death . . . emotionally and spiritually. What's the one thing we're all searching for that can bring peace to our minds and healing to our lives and bodies? What would you say if I told you that you already know? You just don't *know* that you know. It's also right where you are, right now and you can use it any time you choose to heal any part of your life. It's the most powerful force in existence and can create changes in your life that could only be described as miraculous.

IT'S LOVE. SELF-LOVE.

I can imagine what you must be thinking. You've read all "those" books before. The problem with self-love is that it's become such a talk-show, self-help buzzword over the years that it's almost a cliché. Make no mistake: Real self-love is more than an ambiguous, ethereal concept. It's a tangible, evolutionary force that can transform your entire life far beyond anything you can imagine. There's a reason the first four letters of "evolution" spell "love." You don't see it at first because the letters are backwards. It's hidden. Evolution and change are grounded in love because they move us *forward* in life, but the immediate benefits can be hidden from us because we don't know how to look deeper. Throughout this book, you'll read how self-love dramatically changes lives, including my own. This book was written to help you enact the same profound change in your life.

What does it mean to love yourself? How do you "do" it? Most of us get excited when we learn about the power of self-love and are ready to get busy "loving" our dreams into reality. So, we run out and buy ourselves a bouquet of flowers or soak in a special bubble bath that night . . . and wonder why nothing happens. We become disillusioned because no one told us that self-love is an act of "being"—not doing. You'll come to understand that the key to self-love requires far less action than you think. It's a *natural progression* that automatically happens once you understand two other key emotions. The real healing solution to all the problems of your life . . . of the human race is really quite simple. Notice I didn't say easy. Actually, it is easy, but deceptively so because we overcomplicate the matter, as we do most things in life. It's the missing piece of the puzzle that's always been hidden in plain sight.

Renowned author and metaphysical teacher Louise Hay has counseled thousands of people over the years. She has repeatedly said that no matter what someone might have been dealing with at the time, whether it was a lack of money, relationship turmoil, or health problems, she only worked on one issue with them: loving the self. In fact, she healed her own body by understanding these very concepts. As a physician, I can claim the same experience. I have seen thousands of patients throughout my years in practice and can attest to the fact that all healing, whether it's from something minor or life-threatening, is based in self-love. Not only do those who live these concepts heal, but they heal better and faster.

This is a book for everyone, no matter what challenge they face. It doesn't matter if the struggle is with alcohol, drug abuse, relationship problems, or health concerns. Our inner turmoil takes on any number of manifestations that are unique to the individual, but there is only ever one cause and cure: the lack of and return to self-love.

I've chosen to focus this book, however, on those dealing with weight problems. There is a specific reason for this. If you happen to pass someone on the street you might never know they're dealing with something like diabetes or perhaps a sex addiction. They can "pass" in daily life. They can go about their business, blend in perfectly with society, and no one is wise to the inner battle they're waging. Those who deal with weight problems, however, are forced to move about the world in a body that glaringly puts their emotional pain on display every single day. In addition to dealing with the initial pain that caused the weight gain in the first place, they now have the added humiliation of trying to function in a world that has no compassion for anyone who is mildly overweight, not to mention obese. A study published in *Obesity: A Research Journal* in 2008 showed that in the decade between 1996 and 2006, discrimination against obese Americans increased by 66%.[1] A review of data from the *National Survey of Midlife Development in the United States* showed that overweight, obese, and severely obese people are 12, 37, and 100 times more likely to experience discrimination in employment.[2]

With so much animosity toward people with weight challenges, you might think the one person they could find compassion from is their healthcare provider. After all, we *are* in the healing business, which requires a certain amount of empathy, right? Shockingly, that's not so. A study of over 620 primary care physicians showed that more than 50% viewed obese patients as awkward, ugly, and noncompliant. One third of the respondents said obese patients lacked willpower and were lazy. The majority also felt obesity was simply a "behavioral problem" brought on by overeating and lack of exercise.[3] Nurses don't fare much better. A study published by the *Journal of Advanced Nursing* found that nurses regularly expressed biased attitudes toward obese patients, often engaging in stereotypes that they were lazy, noncompliant, and lacked self-control.[4]

If these "compassionate" professionals feel this way, you can imagine what the average man on the street thinks about people with weight challenges. What no one seems to realize is that, while there are many manifestations of problems in our lives, there is only one cause: a lack of love. The problem overweight people face is that others can *see* that manifestation and then, they are judged by it. So in reality, we're all dealing with the same issue. We all have the *same* problem. As I said, we're all hungry.

Don't make the mistake of thinking this is a "diet" or "weight loss" program. You'll be doing yourself a great disservice. In fact, there probably isn't anything new I could tell you about carbs, calorie counting, metabolic rates, or exercise that you don't already know. Most overweight people will tell you they've read so many of those books that they've earned an informal Ph.D. in nutrition. That's not really a joke. I know people who have dieted for so many years they can tell you exactly how many calories are in a single blueberry and how much aerobic activity is needed to burn off a slice of cheese. With that kind of knowledge, why would anyone still struggle with weight? It's because losing weight is not a food issue. It's a love issue. Trying to lose weight by focusing on food is like trying to quit smoking by focusing on cigarettes. How does that make sense?

All those statistics about nutrition and exercise are just intellectual knowledge. It's absolutely useless when you're dealing with an emotional issue. Intellect involves the brain and is great for balancing your checkbook. Emotion, however, resides within the heart and involves much deeper concepts, such as compassion and intuition. It leads us in directions that don't immediately make sense, but somehow we just *know* it's the right thing to do. It's the difference between trying to figure something out and *feeling* something out.

You might think the power of love or the heart is just a figure of speech. How many times have you heard someone say, "Listen to your heart," or ask, "What does your heart tell you?" Did you take them seriously? Were they just being kind or does the heart really have its own power and intelligence? You may be surprised to know that a study done by the Institute of HeartMath found that the bioelectromagnetic field of the heart is 5,000 times stronger than that of the brain, and can actually be measured radiating several feet out from the body.[5]

Anytime we experience what we perceive as a "problem" in our lives, we have become separated from our sacred selves. A problem is simply a call to return to our authentic nature. The journey back to love is a journey back to God and to remembering who you really are. Because this is very much a sacred journey, I've based this program on a 40-day plan. I chose 40 days because, across all the major faiths and belief systems, the number 40 carries great significance. It represents overcoming adversity, a return from being outcast, cleansing, and a coming-of-age wisdom.

In the Christian tradition, Christ survived 40 days of fasting and temptation in the desert, while Noah emerged from the great flood after 40 days and nights. For 40 years, the Jews wandered in the desert in search of the Promised Land. In Islam, 40 is the number of change and reconciliation, while Mohammed received his calling at the age of 40. The list goes on and on.

The program also includes 40 exercises, one for each day. Unlike "talk therapy," these are not intellectual in nature, requiring you to "figure" something out. The exercises are *active* and require real participation on your part, because life is a *sensorial* experience, not an intellectual evaluation. Your heart and body also have their own language, and in order to speak it, we'll need to bypass that "thinking" watcher-at-the-gate: your brain. The exercises are fun, enlightening, and challenging, designed to reveal your greatest gifts. So, have courage and persistence as you move through them, because the greatest treasure is always hidden in the dark.

There is a nutritional suggestion for each day of the program, but don't let that intimidate you. It is merely a suggestion. The same goes for exercise. I've not addressed the issue here, but it's always good to have some type of physical activity going. You should consult your own doctor if you have something in mind. I would just suggest that it be something organic and fun, such as dancing, so that this program never seems like a chore or "work." Your enthusiasm for the program is essential to its success.

I've not directly addressed exercise because I do not believe that it is the primary issue in permanent weight loss. If you ask bodybuilders how they achieve such an amazing physique, they will tell you that 90% of the real work is *not* in the gym. It's what they put in their mouths. In regard to weight loss, I say that 90% of the success comes from what you put in your heart/mind, and that diet and exercise only count for about 10%. I think that's made quite clear when you see how many people can eat whatever they want, rarely exercise, and maintain perfect weight. They're doing something right, and it's not in the kitchen or the gym.

So I want you to begin this book at the end: your end. How do you see yourself at the ideal weight? What do you want to look like? What kind of clothes do you want to wear? What kind of activities would you be doing at your ideal weight? Take that image and hold onto it. Carry it with you in the back of your mind for the next 40 days. We'll discuss how powerful intention and visualizations are, but for now, I want you to set your destination in mind. Just know you're like the famous tightrope walker, Philippe Petit, who walked between the World Trade Center twin towers in 1974. To make such a seemingly "impossible" journey, he had to be completely conscious of where he was on the wire at every moment, but never once take his eyes off his destination. He had an intention of where he was going, but always knew where he was in relation to it. His *intention* was the goal, while his *attention* was perfectly present in the moment with each new step.

Just by making this decision, you set in motion an event that will create a positive ripple effect in your life. In applied mathematics, the Law of Sensitive Dependence on Initial Conditions states that even a *tiny change* over the course of time will result in a *profound* effect. Think of it this way: If a ship, leaving New York headed for Great Britain, veers its direction by just one degree, it will eventually find itself hundreds of miles off-course, in a completely different destination! That's the compounding power of simply making a decision, and then the next decision, and so on.

I want you to know that you are safe within these pages, and most importantly, that you are loved. You are reading a book from someone who has "been there" and my personal journey has influenced this entire program. All your power is right here, right NOW. You will get there because this is a book about *creating*, not coping, *transcending* and not trying, *healing* instead of heartbreak, and *solutions* instead of sales pitches. Most importantly, it's a book about love—your love.

Every patient who enters my office crosses a huge mat that reads, "Regardless of where I have been, I choose to step into my loving." Say that to yourself now . . . out loud. Feel the freedom in it as we take that first step now, together.

CHAPTER I

THE REAL YOU

*"We are not human beings having a spiritual experience.
We are spiritual beings having a human experience."*
—Pierre Tielhard de Chardin, *French philosopher*

"It takes courage to grow up and be who you really are."
—e.e. cummings, *poet*

*"How many cares one loses when one decides
not to be something, but to be someone."*

—Coco Chanel, *fashion designer*

From the time anyone begins a struggle with weight, their entire life revolves around their physical body. *Will I crowd the people beside me at this restaurant table? I can't order what I really want or the waiter will judge me. I won't ask for the help I need from this sales clerk because she'll look at me like I have no business in this clothing boutique. I'll do my grocery shopping after 10:00 p.m. when fewer people are in the store so they won't stare in my cart.* These kinds of thoughts often become a tidal wave in the minds of overweight people when they engage in simple, everyday tasks. The most basic daily activities become an immense amount of work, and even cause panic in some who feel they must constantly compensate for their weight.

Because they feel out of control with regard to their weight, some of these people revert to obsessing over their physical appearance. They say it's about battling stereotypes that overweight people are frumpy or unhygienic. So, they dress to the nines every day just to run errands or take their dogs to the park. These are men and women who won't leave the house unless perfectly coiffed and coordinated, and yet, I've seen actresses in line at the bank with rollers in their hair. The pressure to look squeaky clean, beautiful, and perfect all the time is crushing. Even though they may be the best-looking, best-dressed person at the gas station or post office, they're still thinking, *"No one understands. If they only knew who I really was."*

What's really going on? Everyone wants to look good, but such self-imposed pressure goes beyond disproving stereotypes. It's an attempt to present oneself as "worthy" enough just to participate in the same daily activities as everyone else. You don't need anyone's permission to live in the world. You're worthy right now. I know you see the skinny version of yourself trapped inside your body as the *real* you. Is it? You might just be surprised.

UNDER/STANDING YOUR WORLD

Ironically, one of the least-understood words in the English language is "understand." When you're going through a difficult time and someone says, "I understand," can they ever really know what it's like for you without having experienced the same situation? The best they could ever do is to make an educated guess. We're constantly saying we understand all sorts of things in life. In reality, we're filtering them through our assumptions of how a situation might be, as opposed to basing our idea on real experience.

To understand something means that we have chosen to *stand under* a commonly accepted idea of what something is really about. It means to accept as true the collective consensus or mass majority's belief of any particular subject. Although we may not have the exact answer to a particular issue or problem, we easily sign onto the most widely-accepted explanation. It has to be the right answer; otherwise so many people wouldn't believe it, right?

Healing from experiences such as body dysmorphia, weight gain, and their underlying spiritual causes ignites deeper realizations about our true identity, purpose, and power that significantly alter what we once thought we understood about ourselves and our universe. It requires the courage to step out from under some of the most widely-accepted belief systems and forge a healing path that is uniquely your own. Challenging beliefs you've held your entire life can be unsettling, but also liberating.

Take a quick inventory of some of the beliefs you hold, from weight and nutrition to religion or even politics. *Republicans help only the rich. Democrats love to raise taxes. My religion is the one true faith. My whole family is overweight, therefore I'm genetically doomed.* If you look closely, you'll find that most of what you believe you've either heard from someone else or read somewhere. That means you've decided to stand under a consensus/mass majority idea about something with little or no real proof (experience) to base it on. It's shocking how much we choose to believe and ultimately guide our lives by simply because someone else "said so." More often than not, these erroneous beliefs end up severely limiting our potential and, ultimately, our lives. It's time to begin challenging what you once thought you understood about your world, beginning with yourself.

AN I-OPENING EXPERIENCE

When we find that most of our deeply-held lifelong beliefs about ourselves simply aren't true, we're left standing under a whole new paradigm of who we are and how the universe works. It's the exhilarating realization that not only are we NOT who we thought we were, but we CAN be everything we've always wanted to be. Our potential and possibilities are truly endless. It's more than just stepping outside the box. It's obliterating the box itself.

It's the paradigm shift I refer to as an I-volution. It's a profound awakening from the small (i) of who you thought you were: the ego-centered, hurting, helpless victim that clung to every lie about your beauty, size, earning potential, and relationship possibilities that anyone ever told you, and expanding into the confident, beautiful, courageous, and successful person you really are: the big (I). Before there can be any *evolution* in the outer conditions of our lives, there must be an *involution*, and involution begins with I.

Keeping it Simple

Nearly the entire self-help industry is convinced that life is hard. Countless books and therapists will tell you that most real and lasting change usually takes a lifetime to achieve. Unfortunately, many people have chosen that understanding and live their lives with the expectation that everything is a constant struggle. How many times have you heard someone say, *"Why does life have to be so hard?"* or, *"No matter how hard I try, nothing changes"*? Even in a lighter, more comical way, we've accepted this notion. You might hear someone laugh after something negative happens and say, *"Yeah, life's a bitch and then you die."* We've given away our personal power, and now the idea that life is a constant uphill battle has permeated our culture.

As complex as our individual lives may be at times, I say the true essence of life is really quite simple. Whenever you're overwhelmed by problems in your life and feel like everything is out of control, stop a moment and look to nature. Grass doesn't struggle to grow. Summer doesn't refuse to give way to autumn. Rivers always flow along the path of *least resistance*. No matter where your life is at this moment, you can be assured that everything *is* in balance. The universe in which you live, and play an interactive part, is an orderly place. Science has actually proven this to be true.

Sacred geometry is an historical, studied discipline that examines the patterns that occur in nature. It explains how honeybees can replicate thousands of perfectly identical hexagonal cells in their hive, and why the dimensions of every single snowflake are perfectly symmetrical and mathematically precise. The leaves of plants and trees even grow outward from their center at geometrically predictable intervals based on a formula known as the Fibonacci sequence. You can find these same mathematical relations in every great piece of art, architecture and music throughout history. You can see evidence of it in your own body, as it determines the ratio of your arm length to your leg length and the spatial relationship of your facial features. You don't have to be a mathematician to see that order rules our world and that life is anything but random.

OUTSIDE IN

So if everything is in balance and life is much simpler than we think, how does it appear to get so complicated? If life is really simple, then the answer to that question must be a simple one. In order to answer it, however we must go back and revisit that notion of *who* or *what* it is that you think you are.

Even people who don't deal with a weight challenge tend to be overly fixated on their physical bodies. From the fitness and bodybuilding craze to weight loss reality TV shows and the obsession with plastic surgery, people seem to be spending nearly all their energy (and money) on how they look. The next time you're waiting in the grocery store checkout line, count how many headlines you see on the magazine covers that have anything to do with the body. I counted 29 on seven covers! Turn on your TV any time after 10:00 p.m. and half the channels are promoting gadgets that will tighten and tone "this" or creams that will lift and smooth "that." The truth is; we've got it backwards. We're working life from the outside in, when it's really an inside job to begin with.

WIDE OPEN SPACES

This body that we've become so obsessed with, that we think is so solid, permanent and concrete, that we think is "me" . . . really isn't. Let's take an imaginary super-powered microscope and journey inside the body. First, we see organ systems and then individual organs. We'll focus on the heart for this example. As we look deeper, we see the heart is made of tissue and that tissue is composed of cells. Journeying inside the cells we discover they're made of molecules. Inside the molecules, we see individual atoms. Amazingly, the **vast majority** of the inside of these atoms is *nothing* . . . but open space. There's literally nothing there except for a few protons, neutrons, and electrons. Sources vary in number, but it's basically accepted that the human body is made up of somewhere between 50 and 100 trillion cells, and the story is the same for every single one of them. In fact, when you add the sum of their parts, your body is *far, far* more open space and emptiness than anything else. As scientists continue to look closer into the body, they're finding that it is far less material-based and much more *frequency-based* than we've ever thought before. It was Nobel Prize-winning quantum physicist Werner Heisenberg who said, *"Atoms or elementary particles themselves are not real; they form a world of potentialities or possibilities rather than one of things or facts."*

12

Scientists have intuitively known the essence of life is simple and have spent the better part of the last century looking for one theory that can explain why things come into being. We've long known of many laws that govern the universe, such as Isaac Newton's law of gravity, Albert Einstein's theory of relativity, or James Clerk Maxwell's theory of electromagnetism. What we didn't have was one rule that tied them all together in a simple explanation of life.

It was in a conference at the University of Southern California in 1995 that physicist Edward Witten of the Institute for Advanced Study stunned the world when he presented his M-Theory. Building upon the work of physicist Leonard Susskind of Stanford University in the 1970s, Witten's M-Theory or String Theory was both shocking and beautiful. It said that physical matter isn't truly real. Everything, whether it's a tree, a butterfly, or your body is all made up of exactly the same thing: infinitesimally small vibrating strands of energy.[6] What makes them appear in different forms is simply the rate or frequency at which those strands are vibrating. Not only was this discovery a boon for science, but it gave credence to the mystics and sages who have said for millennia that we are all ONE and that everything is *the same thing*.

THOUGHTS BECOME THINGS

So if everything is just energy in vibration, what controls the rate of that vibration to make you, you? The answer is: your thoughts. Thought waves have their own frequency much like gamma waves, radio waves, or microwaves, and they are the conductors that mold the very energy that makes up your body. In fact, thought waves are so powerful that they don't just create your body, but every situation you bring into your life. This includes your finances, relationships, health, and weight. Thoughts *really do* become things. In fact, thoughts are so powerful it's the reason all sciences, including medicine, conduct double blind studies for research. It's been known for quite some time that if a researcher expects a certain result from an experiment he's conducting; his thoughts and expectations *will* affect the outcome.

Authors Robert Monroe and William Buhlman have studied this phenomenon in people who had near death or out of body experiences for decades. Their subjects said that while "out of body" their thoughts created objects and circumstances in their environment instantaneously. The same principle applies to those of us in this slightly denser world of "physical" matter. The manifestation of our thoughts just takes a bit longer. Buhlman says in his book, *Adventures Beyond the Body*, "Once you fully recognize the power of your thoughts, you will never again create or hold a negative or destructive image in your mind. Negative and self-limiting thoughts are the real enemy we must face."[7] This gives real meaning to the old saying, "Be careful what you wish for. You might get it."

CONSTANT CHANGE

The only thing constant is change. How many times have you heard that? Now we know it's true. The only thing constant is the ever-flowing energy soup that we all reside in that's forever changing form based on the rate of vibration it takes on. Everything in life is built on a continuous cycle of regeneration and renewal. Winter always turns to Spring. The moon gives way to the sun each morning. Earth that was charred and barren from wildfires soon sprouts green with life again. While it may look the same to you year to year, even your body is in a constant state of renewal.

Everyone knows hair, skin and fingernail cells continue to grow throughout life. What science is finally discovering is that virtually *every cell* in your body is renewed on a regular basis. This includes cells for organs for which regeneration was once thought impossible, such as the brain and heart. A study recently performed at the Karolinska Institute in Stockholm, Sweden, has proven that human beings actually regenerate heart cells throughout their entire life span.[8] Radioactive isotope studies are showing that you get a new stomach lining every five days and a brand-new skeletal system in about three months. In fact, in less than two years we replace nearly 98% of all the cells in our entire body. In just over two years we have a *brand-new body.*[9] Even the body you had when you started reading this book isn't the same one, on a cellular level, that you have at this moment. The very bedrock of our universe is this amazing principle of renewal and change. The universe *wants* your body to change. It's been designed specifically for that very purpose. By its own rules, the universe is on your side when it comes to weight loss. It WANTS you to be at a healthy weight and has given you every advantage and tool to accomplish that.

THE DRIVER'S SEAT

If all the cards are on your side, why is weight loss so difficult? I'm sure you've heard the phrase, "The more things change, the more they stay the same." Our concept of things staying the same isn't really accurate, based on what we've just learned. It's more like they're repeating themselves. We've gotten stuck in a mental loop by continuing to think in a certain way about our bodies that puts out a negative vibration. If the instructions we keep giving the energy inside our cells is, "I'm fat, unattractive, and worthless," then it's going to continue to reconfigure itself to match those instructions. So your body is, in fact, constantly changing. Your thoughts, however, just keep changing it back into the same form over and over again, so it only looks like there is no movement. You truly are in the driver's seat when it comes to your body. You've just been driving down the same road for too long!

No matter where you look, science has now begun to prove what the ancient mystics and sages have known for thousands of years. From the ancient Emerald Tablets of Hermes that begin with the famous phrase, "As Above, So Below" to the more common proverb of "Mind Over Matter," it's virtually indisputable that we create our entire life experience by the vibrations we're emitting that correspond to the thoughts we're habitually thinking.

ATTRACTION IN ACTION

Nikola Tesla, the inventor of the radio, once said, "If you want to find the secrets of the universe, think in terms of energy, frequency, and vibration." It's through vibration that we attract every object, person, and situation into our lives. Philosophers have called it the Law of Attraction. Theologians referred to it by saying, "You reap what you sow." It's all the same principle. We bring back to us everything we put out into the world. That includes every action we take and thinking a thought *is* taking an action—a very big one, because life isn't so much dynamic as it is *magnetic*. We draw things to us. Life doesn't happen to us. It happens *through* us. You may remember your grandmother saying to you, "God helps those who help themselves." That wasn't a metaphor. She was right.

One of the most crucial ways you can begin to help yourself lose weight is by changing your thoughts about it. Remember, whatever you put out into the universe comes back to you. The universe is *affirmative*, not negative. It trusts that **you** know what's best for you and you do! You're the expert on you. Naturally, if you're going about your day thinking, *"I want to lose weight"* or *"I wish I could lose weight,"* the focus is on your weight and that's all the universe is hearing: *weight*. By the divine law of the universe, that's what will come back to you—more weight. If you're thinking, *"I don't want to be fat,"* you're not speaking thinness to the universe. It hears *"fat"* and that's what you get.

ATTENTION & DIRECTION

Whatever you focus on expands in your life because that's where you're directing your energy. Because the universe is affirmative by nature, don't think about losing weight through this program because that's what you'll get, weight. That's why scale-oriented weigh-in based diets never work . . . at least not long term. Think about this as a journey to finding love. Detaching yourself from any reference to your physical weight is extremely important to getting the most out of this program.

Detachment to the outcome is so important because it lifts the pressure off of having to achieve a specific goal by a specific time. I'm sure you know what deadlines and "goals" can do to your weight loss motivations. *"I've **got** to lose 20 pounds before my wedding."* Detaching from all those requirements gives you permission to enjoy the journey on the way to a destination that will reveal itself once you get there. Here's an example. Have you ever had this type of experience? You've been invited to go bowling with friends. You don't really bowl but you decide to tag along. While there, you're laughing with your friends, not paying any attention to the game. Suddenly, you bowl a strike, then another and then another! The less you "try" the better you do while your bowling friends are stunned at your effortless success. That's the kind of mental space you need to be in for successful weight loss. Have fun. Enjoy the discovery. Learn new things about yourself. Get excited. Just do not focus on trying to lose weight.

The most valuable commodity you can ever give anyone or anything is your attention, because it will eventually be replicated in your life experience. Here's a fun experiment to demonstrate the power of your attention: Pretend you're in the market for a new car. Choose one that you like. Look it up online. A lot of manufacturer websites have interactive features where you can actually design your car right down to the color and wheel rims. Have fun with it. See yourself driving the new car. Do this for a few days and watch what happens. Suddenly, you'll start seeing that exact type of car all over town. You'll park next to one at the grocery store. You'll notice one at a stop light. You'll see five TV commercials for the same car in a couple of hours. That's the power and speed at which the universe works though your attention, and it's time to start putting it to work on what you want . . . and deserve.

REALITY CHECK... THE REAL YOU

✓ No matter what problem anyone may have, be it health issues, relationship problems, financial trouble or weight challenges; it all stems from a lack of love—self-love.

✓ Self-love is an act of being—not "doing."

✓ A return to self-love allows all areas of our lives to fall naturally into place without struggle.

✓ The bioelectromagnetic field of the heart is 5,000 times stronger than the brain. That's the power of the healing force of love!

✓ Permanent weight loss is a love issue—not a food issue.

✓ Losing weight permanently means challenging the erroneous beliefs we've collected from other sources regarding what he thought we "understood" about ourselves.

✓ Challenging old beliefs is the first step to having a true I-opening experience.

✓ You are NOT your body! Your body and everything else in the universe is just energy in vibration.

✓ You control your vibration and create your entire world through your thoughts.

✓ What you're focusing on in your life is expanding right now.

✓ We can change our lives by changing our thoughts.

FOOD FOR THOUGHT

On the Flipside

Have you been thinking in reverse and putting your attention on the things you don't want? Reframe those thoughts and start looking at them from the other side. Turn them into affirmative statements about what you DO want, so you can begin to bring these things into your life. Take a moment to write down some common beliefs you have about weight that affect different areas of your life. Try flipping these around to more positive statements about what you DO want. Holding onto these new thoughts is the first step to creating real change. Remember, the universe is *affirmative* and gives you whatever you're focusing on!

Examples:

Weight: I DON'T want to be fat anymore.
I want to be my ideal weight, healthy and happy.

Relationships: I DON'T want to face people's cruelty. I'll stay home alone.
I'd love to meet kind people who respect me for who I am.

Family: I DON'T want my mother to keep pressuring me to lose weight.
I would like my mother to understand me.

Weight: _____

_____

Relationships: _____

_____

Family:_____

_____

Romance: _____

_____

Employment: _____

_____

Clothes:_____

_____

Food:_____

_____

CHAPTER 2

BELIEVE IT OR NOT

~~~

Do not believe in anything simply because you have heard it.

*Do not believe anything simply because
it is spoken of and rumored by many.*

*Do not believe anything simply because
it is written in your religious books.*

*Do not believe anything merely on
the authority of your teachers and elders.*

*Do not believe in traditions simply because
they have been handed down for many generations.*

*But after observation and analysis, when you find
anything agrees with reason and is conducive
to the benefit of one and all, then accept it and live by it.*

—**Buddha**, *founder of Buddhism*

We know that we create our bodies and, in fact, our entire life circumstances by the vibrations we're sending out into the Universe based on what we're thinking. Even so, you might ask, *"But I don't think about my weight 100% of the day. Why doesn't anything change for me, even just a little bit?"* That's because your personal energy vibration arises mostly from thoughts you don't even realize you're thinking. They're thoughts most of us just take for granted. They're our beliefs. Everything in our lives, including our weight, manifests not from what we *wish* or *hope* for, but what we deeply *believe* about ourselves.

What do you believe and why do you believe it? It's amazing how rarely we ask ourselves those questions about the ideas on which we base our very lives. Most people probably can't tell you where they picked up some of their most fervent beliefs. All they know is that they've believed them for so long that they've just become a part of them. Not understanding what you believe, and more importantly, *why* you believe it, is like living your life on autopilot. "Just believing" in something is the reason we have so much chaos in our individual and collective world.

Just Because

How many times growing up did your parents tell you to do something and you simply asked, "*Why?*" The usual, parent-approved response is almost always, "*Because.*" You asked again, "*Why?*" They said, "*Just because.*" Clearly, that explained nothing, so you asked again, "*Why?*" They sternly added, "*Because I said so.*" Still not good enough, you pressed your luck, "*But* **why?**" The game ended when they snapped back, "*Because I'm the grown-up. That's why. Now just do it.*"

Even the most well-meaning parents misinterpret this kind of behavior as questioning their authority. What they don't realize is that dampening a child's inquisitiveness is actually shutting down their critical thinking process. It teaches them that asking questions is disrespectful at best, and at worst, invites punishment. So as children, we acquiesce and learn to stop asking the single most important question in our lives, "*Why?*" As a result, we simply begin to accept ideas about ourselves and our world strictly at face value, without filtering them through any kind of instinct, intuition, or just a healthy dose of common sense. It seems like the right thing to do because it comes from people we trust.

The Parent Trap

Most of our beliefs about ourselves and our world come from our parents. Any authority figure in a child's life, such as a teacher or clergyman, can make significant contributions, too. These beliefs are usually set in our minds by the age of five or so. That's the age psychologists believe the development of the human psyche, which gives rise to our individual personality, is complete. During that time, virtually all our interaction is with our parents. As children, we see our parents as infallible protectors and take their word as absolute truth. Why shouldn't we? They're supposed to know what's best for us. The problem arises when we have parents who are less than ideal, and that's nearly everyone. When you look at the staggering number of people who are in 12-step programs, psychotherapy, substance abuse rehabilitation, or even prison, you'll see the vast majority of us were not growing up inside a TV sitcom household . . . and these are just the people who *know* there's something amiss in their lives. An even larger number still have no idea why they're on their fourth marriage, third bankruptcy, or twentieth diet. It all stems from unconscious beliefs that are driving behaviors acquired much earlier in life.

CRIMES OF OMISSION

While it's easier to see how extreme physical, verbal, or sexual abuse as children affects us in our adult lives, most parental offenses aren't crimes of commission, but rather ones of omission. What a parent *doesn't do* can be as powerful and affecting as what they choose to do in raising a child. When we grow up with parents who dismiss us, ignore us, or are physically and emotionally unavailable, we assume we are unloved. In psychology, this kind of parental emotional detachment is known as proximal abandonment. If we are unworthy of the love of the most important people in our lives, then it's easy to believe in a God that does not love us. Ultimately, we end up not loving ourselves either because we simply don't know *how* to.

As the most powerful and intelligent creature that's ever walked the face of the Earth, man begins his life as one of the most vulnerable. While fish, reptiles, and even insects are born ready to immediately begin their self-sufficient lives, a human child can't even hold its own head up. Once it exits the birth canal, a baby must immediately *learn* to breathe air. Even with this most basic of biological functions we require help as the doctor gives a baby a pat on the bottom to induce a cry and expand its thoracic cavity. As infants, we must be provided with and taught virtually everything. That includes love. Yes, we *learn* how to love. It must be taught to us and we learn it by experiencing it.

I was having a consultation with a patient about what experiences might be contributing to his specific health issues. When the subject of his mother came up, he told me, *"I know my mother loved me because she would make my favorite pancakes for breakfast."* While he could intellectualize that idea as an adult, it's not what his subconscious belief was about his mother, who was always away working in his early years. Children think literally, and a pancake is just a pancake. That's all. To experience love, a child needs to *feel* it. Feeling is the door to the subconscious and where most of our beliefs are stored. When a child is held, touched, hugged, played with, tickled, or rocked to sleep, words are unnecessary. The message is clear. They are safe, secure, and most of all, loved.

When we are loved, then we can recognize what love is and provide it to ourselves and others. It's the foundation of all self-esteem and self-confidence that leads to personal achievement. Without it, we go through life with beliefs such as: *I'm unlovable. I don't deserve love. I'm not enough. There must be something wrong with me.* When we don't know how to love ourselves, we can't love others properly. At its most extreme, it can lead to criminal anti-social behavior, and those who have no conscience or cannot feel empathy for another human being. At the other end of the spectrum, it could be someone who's had a long string of unsuccessful relationships because they're emotionally unavailable to their partners.

JUST THE BASICS

In any case, this love shortage cuts across the entire socioeconomic spectrum. I've seen just as many patients from traditionally "dysfunctional" households as those whose parents *"loved me through the MasterCard."* So many times, parents are shocked by the way their adult children feel because they provided them with the "best" of everything growing up and, therefore, assume they have no right to feel the way they do. The mistake most parents make is that they provide just the basics for children: food, shelter, and clothing. It doesn't matter if it's a mansion or a one-bedroom apartment. As long as they provide these necessities and don't harm the children in any way, most feel the rest of the rearing process will take care of itself. That simply isn't so.

The respected psychologist Abraham Maslow said that all human beings have the ability and right to reach their highest creative potential, which he called Self-Actualization. To reach that point, he said that a human being must be provided with specific needs throughout his life. In order to advance to the next level of development, he must

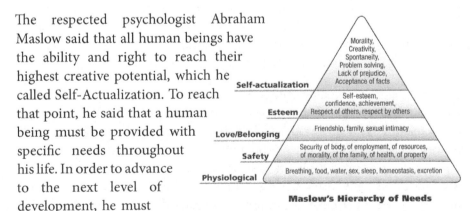

have received the essential needs of the one before it. For example, you can't have a sense of safety at Level 2 if you don't at least have proper food, shelter, and clothing in Level 1. You can see that all self-esteem and achievement is built upon the sense of love, intimacy, and belonging that a child should have received at Level 3. By providing our children with just their material needs, we're doing the absolute *minimum* at the most important job we'll ever have in our lives. We're also teaching them that the minimum is all they deserve.

KNOW BETTER, DO BETTER

Although our parents contribute heavily to our internal beliefs, it doesn't mean that we get to blame them for the mistakes we make through our entire lives. Because *we* create our own lives moment by moment through the choices we make, based on the beliefs we hold, we have to take full responsibility for our experiences. No one else gets to think for you. Only *you* choose the thoughts that fill your attention. That's wonderful! That's the beauty of free will. You get to choose in each moment the thoughts you want to focus on, and what you focus on expands in your life. If we blame others for our mistakes, that means we believe we are victims and don't have the power to change anything because "they" did "this" to me and they're "in control." In order to change our lives, we must accept **full responsibility** that only we created them in their current condition based on the beliefs we're choosing. The payoff for accepting full responsibility is the awareness that you can use this same power to re-create your life in a way that serves you. You cannot begin to change your life until you understand that total responsibility and total power are two sides of the same coin.

This doesn't mean we have to excuse parents for bad decisions. Yes, many parents make terrible mistakes when rearing their children, but it's essential to know that they did the best they could at the time with the knowledge they had. A mother who takes her daughter to six different weight loss clinics before she's even out of high school doesn't realize the message she's sending. When she says, *"Sweetheart, you look beautiful in your prom dress but you'll look gorgeous when you lose ten more pounds,"* she doesn't realize the seed she's planting in her child's mind. Even in situations that were violent or neglectful, we need to realize that our parents didn't know how to process the violence and neglect they experienced and so passed the pain onto us. Anyone who's hurting someone else is *always* in a great deal of pain. Pain only begets pain. When we see that, we can have compassion for our parents and move toward forgiveness.

Sometimes, our pain and struggles don't come directly from our parents, but further back in our family line. Psychologist John Bradshaw has done some fantastic work on this subject in his books, including *Family Secrets*.[10] Because we live in an energetic universe that shapes the physical matter we see, anger, resentment, violence, and traumas can create a negative energetic signature that's passed down through generations of a family. This means a life problem you're dealing with today might be due to a cellular energetic imprint from a negative experience your grandmother or perhaps great-grandmother had. Too many times we write multi-generational problems off as "genetic" and surrender to them when, in fact, it's the emotional energy that's driving the genes to manifest themselves in a specific way, as we'll see a bit later.

The idea is to eliminate family secrets. Clear the air and your familial energy. I highly recommend investigating the backgrounds of your parents and extended family members by speaking with them directly or friends who know them. What you discover will probably surprise you. You'll see that their intentions were never to hurt you personally, but rather an unconscious perpetuation of beliefs and patterns they accepted from their own parents. The good news is that, as we make an effort to expose these beliefs, we can change them and break generational patterns. By knowing better, we do better.

Domestic Dynamics

When investigating the origin of your beliefs, it's also important to look at the dynamics within the family itself in addition to the relationships between family members. This is important for those who grew up in seemingly normal homes with good parents, where there was no overt violence or neglect, but can't seem to get to the root of their beliefs.

Perhaps you know one of these "perfect" families. Everyone seems happy and successful except for one "problem" child. Constantly getting into trouble and acting out, it's almost like the child is from a different family. As an adult, they might even end up in jail or addicted to drugs. Too often, we look at our siblings' success and feel we have no right to be sad, depressed, or angry because we all grew up in the same house. If they're doing great, raised by the same parents, then the problem is me. I'm defective in some way.

Before we judge ourselves, it's important to know that anytime a new child comes into a family, the dynamics of how that family functions changes. A stay-at-home mother might have had the luxury of providing loving attention to her first three children, but had to begin working once the fourth child came along. Although we view these kinds of experiences with a sort of matter-of-factness, they can create profound differences in the rearing experiences of children, even within the same family.

JUST DESSERTS

Most people believe that life isn't fair. How could it be when there are so many good people starving, getting into accidents, and having all sorts of misfortune befall them? I believe that life is perfectly fair. Remember that we live in a universe of order that is balanced to the most exacting degree. The Earth is tilted on its axis at the most precise angle to create our seasonal climates and sustain life on the planet. If this tilted angle were shifted by even a fraction of a degree, the planet would fall out of orbit and go hurtling off into space. When bad things happen to good people, it's not because there is some "evil" force that's targeted them for troubles. We already know there is only ONE substance, ONE force in the universe that creates anything. So if there's only ONE power, how could it be good AND evil? The answer is not in the power itself, but in how each of us uses it in our lives. Fire is neither good nor bad. It simply is. If we use it to cook our dinner, we perceive it as a good thing. If we burn our hand in the process, then it's a "bad" thing.

We each have the ability to re-create our lives on a daily basis by managing our personal thought energy that arises from our beliefs. If something negative is happening in your life, it's time to look internally and examine how you are attracting these circumstances into your life based on your beliefs about yourself. As I've said, these beliefs are rooted in our early upbringing and define what we feel we deserve in life.

You performed an exercise in chapter one to clarify what it is that you *want* in life, but do you know what you believe you *deserve* in these same areas? If you're not sure, look in your checkbook and around your home. That's what you believe you deserve financially. Look at the quality of your relationships. That's what you believe you deserve emotionally. Look at your weight and health. That's what you believe you deserve physically. Remember that your subconscious is always working to prove you're right, to establish order in your life or personal universe so you don't think you're crazy. In the middle of seeming chaos, your life makes perfect sense. Everything is perfectly in balance based on what you believe you deserve, and we will only ever experience in life what we feel is "normal" for us.

SHORT CHANGE

Has something like this ever happened to you? You win a sum of money through an instant lottery ticket, a raffle, or perhaps you receive it unexpectedly in a birthday card from a relative. Let's say its $500. Two days later, your car breaks down and the bill comes to . . . you guessed it: $500. That happened because somewhere in your belief system you felt you didn't deserve that money, so you had to create a way to get rid of it. It's the same reason why so many lottery winners end up filing for bankruptcy. On an unconscious level, they don't feel they deserve prosperity. In an interview with the *Lincoln Journal Star*, Connecticut financial planner Daryl LePage said:

> *"We know from studies and our own internal research that when new wealth is created in a family, there is a 90-percent probability that all of that wealth will be gone by the third generation. And that's among families who have worked hard for years to achieve success. When people receive sudden wealth, like in a lottery jackpot, the numbers are much worse. [Money] reveals character and magnifies all of the good and bad traits the winners live by."[11]*

This is the same reason we sabotage ourselves in all areas of our lives, especially when we want to lose weight so badly. Logically, someone can clearly say, *"Of course I deserve to lose weight and be healthier,"* and truly mean it, but it's what they believe they **deserve** on a subconscious level that's really driving the process. That's why so many of us fall off the diet wagon only to beat up on ourselves because we didn't do it "right" this time around.

IN THE DETAILS

Not knowing what we really believe we deserve in our lives can be frustrating, especially when everything we don't want keeps showing up. The good news is that the answers are never hidden from us. Because life is a mirror reflecting our inner nature back to us, we only have to look at the external conditions of our lives for clues to uncover the hidden beliefs that limit us. It's simply a matter of awareness; raising our consciousness in the choices we make on a daily basis that create our lives. Life is really just a series of choices. One choice leads to the next, and so on. If we don't like where we're at, we can always make a new choice. Consciousness in the moment is what allows us to make new choices that heal and serve us.

Here's a great exercise I like to call "The Trip." Do your best to visualize this scenario in **as much detail as you can.** You've received a call from your best friend in a neighboring city telling you that she's being honored with a prestigious award at an upcoming celebration. You're very excited for her and say that you'd be happy to attend. The travel day arrives and you board the airplane, eager to see your friend, who you haven't visited in several years. Once you arrive, you check into the hotel and run out shortly afterward to find something to wear to the celebration. That evening, you greet your friend with heartfelt congratulations. She introduces you to a friend who's heard quite a bit about you. You spend the evening chatting and then return to the hotel for the trip home the next morning. **STOP.** Really imagine this experience before reading on.

This sounds like a straightforward experience, right? Let's take a closer look at your "trip." What hotel did you stay in? Was it the Four Seasons, Howard Johnson, or something in between? Where did you buy your outfit for the gala: at a discount department store or a specialty boutique? What kind of outfit did you buy: a designer creation or something off the rack? Was the person you were introduced to attractive and engaging, or did you have a polite, business-like conversation?

When it comes to our lives, it's the subtle energies of our expectations that drive us. They arise from our thoughts based on what we believe we deserve. This exercise probably revealed some interesting things about what you unconsciously feel you deserve in several areas of life. Look deeper, because life is giving us the answers all the time. If you really want to make lasting change in your life, the devil, as they say, is always in the details.

YOUR PERSONAL TRUTH

Once we identify our limiting beliefs, we can challenge them and begin to change them. How do we challenge them? It can be difficult and even unnerving to question beliefs about ourselves and our world that we've used our entire lives to construct our identities. The easiest way is to look at a belief for what it is: *someone else's opinion.* That's all. Just because someone thinks something about you, the world, politics, sex, a specific group of people, or anything else doesn't make it so. It doesn't make it true for you, unless you *choose* to accept it. In the world we live in, everyone has their own truth. It's based on the beliefs they carry that the subtle energies of the universe are constantly rearranging to confirm for them by manifesting corresponding conditions in their life experience. This is why someone can eat a piece of cake and not gain a pound while someone else can have the same slice and it goes "right to the hips." It's because that's what they *believe* even before they take the first bite. The issue isn't how many calories the cake has or how fattening it is. The difference isn't in the cake at all. It's in the mind of the person who's eating it. That's why many people actually lose weight when they stop dieting and focus on food for food's sake: enjoyment, nourishment, and flavor. The idea as to whether a specific food is fattening or not has been completely withdrawn from their consciousness, and thus their body processes food in a different way.

A belief is always someone else's truth about something, but it doesn't have to be *your* truth. Most people who try to foist their beliefs upon us are almost always doing so in an attempt to control us in some way. That's why there is an ancient proverb that says, "He who gives me a belief is my enemy." It's also the same reason the word belief has the word LIE in the middle of it. I also love the saying, "What you think of me is none of my business." Anyone can think anything they want about you, and it has absolutely NO impact on your personal life or well-being because it is impossible for them to think for you. The thoughts and opinions of others have no power over us unless we choose to believe them and make them part of our personal truth.

BELIEFS VS. KNOWNS

A great way to challenge your false beliefs is to compare what you believe with what you KNOW. There's a big difference between believing something and *knowing* something. Knowing something comes from direct physical experience, while believing something is an intellectual choice to see something as true. When you believe something, you have to explain it or justify it to someone else. When you know something, it's self-evident. It needs no explanation. It simply is. Think about your current job. You know what kind of person and skills are required to do your job. Why? Because you've done it. You've had an actual experience, and no amount of debating could convince you otherwise. You know that fire is dangerous. Why? Because you've been burned before. You know that a sense of balance is essential to riding a bicycle. Why? Because you fell down hundreds of times until you developed one. If you take inventory of most of your beliefs in this way, on everything from religion and sex to politics, and especially the ones you have about yourself, you'll be shocked to see how much you *believe* and how little you really *know*.

You might say, *"But I do know that I'm overweight and unattractive. I can look in the mirror and see that."* Really? We've already learned that supposedly material things aren't real. They're simply quantum particles moving around at different frequencies to create the illusion of different objects in life, including your body. It's consciousness or thought energy that's constantly redirecting those particles and telling them how to reshape our personal world every second of our lives. While we've been able to verify this concept scientifically now, the ancient Hindus have understood it for millennia through what they call Maya or the symbolic deity that governs the illusion of the material world. In Sanskrit, it translates to ma (not) and ya (that). To become enlightened in Hinduism is to see beyond the illusion of Maya, and discover that you and the world are *not that* which you perceive with your senses. An artist is not his painting, and you are not that which you've created in your personal world. You are not the creation, but rather the *force* that creates. The same ideology is set forth in the Christian tradition when Christ advises his followers to be "in the world, but not of it." When the creator disentangles himself from identifying with his creation, he then has the power to create *new* things.

So while you're looking in the mirror, ask yourself how much you should really trust your senses when it comes to the illusion of life. If you took everything in life at face value, you might look up into the sky and think the sun is only the size of a grape. You might believe the Earth ends at the horizon line because you see nothing beyond it. The night can seem silent even though animals are emitting thousands of sounds that are outside your hearing range. Interestingly, material objects absorb every color of light in the spectrum *except* for the one they are *not*. That is the color that is reflected back into space. That means an apple is every color *except* red! Realizing that, it's time for a BIG mental paradigm shift.

Playing Catch-Up

From this perspective, we can see that our life situations and our bodies are not *who* we are, just *where* we are at this moment. All of our past beliefs have brought us to the place we are today. The great thing about beliefs is that they can be changed, but we must begin from a place of neutral observation, without judging those who imposed their beliefs on us or ourselves for mistakenly accepting them. It's from this place that our lives immediately begin to change as a result, because we're free from the judgments that used to bog us down. Even though we cannot see it right away, all those quantum particles begin to shift and realign to create new things that match our new, empowered frequency. That's why it's essential to not become discouraged by identifying with what you see in the mirror, especially if it's not changing fast enough for you. It's important to remember that your life situation is the evidence of what *has happened* but NOT what *is happening*. The material world is always playing catch-up with our thoughts, and the length of time it takes to achieve our desires is dependent on how quickly and easily we can get into synch with our new beliefs. Whether it takes a month, a year, or several years to realize our desires is really up to us, but we must stay the course and not give up, because the Universe employs definitive laws that guarantee success if we choose to follow them. The best way to stay on that course is to remember the essential work that's being done for us on an energetic level even though we can't see it, yet. Even the longest winter **must** yield to the spring. The new-thought essayist Robert Bitzer put it best in his treatise *On Spring* when he wrote:

> *"Perhaps this means that winter would be more important than spring. It is in the dormancy of winter that impending life is pulled together, organized and focused. Spring tells you that it has already happened. So does your demonstration. Credit goes to the decision that you made in the silence and to the inner determination that changed your trend of thinking. Spring is the acknowledgment in nature that the silent work of winter was effective. So your demonstration is the acknowledgment in the outer world that your silent creation was real. Spring comes because of what took place in winter."[12]*

REAL SIMPLE

So we live in a universe that's not so much material and concrete as it is an energy soup. Countless elementary particles are dancing around at different frequencies, constantly changing into and out of form, representing all the things we see, hear, taste, touch, and smell as directed by thought energy. As we change our beliefs, the world around us changes. It seems too good to be true, too simple, too basic. There's got to be more, right? Life is so complicated and difficult it couldn't possibly be summed up in something even a child could understand! In fact, it can and it is. Countless philosophies and religious faiths throughout recorded history have said exactly that. Perhaps the most famous confirmation comes from the Christian tradition. Understanding that we create our own heaven or hell here on Earth by the thoughts we choose to shape our lives with, it becomes clear when Christ stated, "Except ye be converted and become as little children, ye shall not enter into the kingdom of heaven."

REALIZE & RELEASE

So, how do you change beliefs? You simply release them. You identify your negative beliefs by examining the conditions your life is returning to you, and through exercises similar to the ones in this chapter. Once you have realized the unconscious beliefs that have been driving your behaviors, you can let them go. It's a process of self-discovery I call *realize and release*.

What if you've spent a lifetime engaging in these negative beliefs about yourself? Won't it take a long time to release those? Won't it be an arduous and painful process? Not really. Remember, we *choose* our beliefs. Once we know better, we can choose something else. The misconception is that personal change takes a long time and is something we must suffer through. That's just not true. You did not come here to learn through suffering. You can learn through joy, too! You came here to live an abundant life through your God-given power of creative thought. It doesn't matter how long you've believed something negative. You can let it go in an instant. That's why half of the word *release* is *EASE*. The real work involved is in uncovering these beliefs. Once they're exposed, you can just let them go. Look at it this way: It can take years to build a massive skyscraper, but a wrecking crew can bring it down in minutes. That's what happens to negative beliefs when they're exposed by the light of truth.

Most people think it takes a massive amount of fuel for the space shuttle to orbit the Earth. It does, but no one realizes that 95% of that fuel is spent right after launch, just to break through Earth's atmosphere. Once it's hundreds of thousands of miles into space, it's smooth sailing. Our goals can look so far away, but we don't realize that the only thing grounding us is the judgments we hold based on our negative perceptions. Once we release those, we're launched into a new life where our desires manifest effortlessly.

Releasing old beliefs is more a matter of *undoing* rather than doing. When we're in the process of applying self-help techniques to improve our lives, we can be our own biggest obstacle by trying to do too much, taking an aggressive approach to "fix" everything at once. This forceful approach almost always backfires, leaving us frustrated because, in the universe, any amount of force is always met with an equal or greater counterforce. That's why surrendering to the process is so important. Releasing the thought *"I'm unattractive"* is far more effective than continuing to believe you're unattractive, but trying to override that mental soundtrack by repeating, affirming, or writing ten thousand times, "I'm beautiful." Your existing false belief will only come rushing back, saying, *"No you're not. No you're not. NO YOU'RE NOT,"* actually *reinforcing* itself. Affirmations have their place in healing, but not before old beliefs are properly realized and released. In this case, it's much more important to begin by realizing you're *not unattractive* than by forcing an idea on yourself that you can't buy into just yet. There's no need to fight old beliefs. It's about making a conscious choice to change your perception of yourself.

All the power to release any belief you choose is in your hands right now, because you're the only one who's been believing it your whole life. It can seem difficult at first, but that's an illusion. There's a reason illusion has the word "ill" in it. Anytime you have an illness or imbalance in your life, there's always an illusion behind it, keeping it going The only thing holding you back is how tightly you've been hanging onto these illusions, how strongly you've used them in the past to define your "identity."

I'm sure you've come home from the grocery store before with more bags than you can handle, but you don't want to make a second trip back to the car. So, you loop the plastic bags through your hands one after the other, until you're so weighted down it's like you're carrying a 100-lb. dumbbell in each hand. With each step, the plastic handles cut deeper and deeper into your hands, but you're determined to make it to the front door. The pain cuts like a knife in the joints of your fingers and the bags feel like they're going to burst, but it's only a few steps more. Once inside, you hoist the bags onto the kitchen counter, and with a sigh of relief, you . . . can't let go of the bags. As hard as you try to open your hands, your fingers are frozen in their death grip around the handles. It's almost like an invisible force has magnetized your hands to the shopping bags. In reality, the only one keeping you hanging on is you. So you use your opposite hand to pry your fingers apart, and once you've released your grip, the sense of relief is overwhelming.

Exposing Core Beliefs

When we expose old subconscious beliefs and challenge their validity, we can release them. Playing the devil's advocate can also be helpful. *How many people have ever said I'm unattractive? Just one. Who? Mother. Oh, well that settles it then. I'm sure the other 6.999 billion people on the planet will be very happy she's spoken for them.* When challenging old beliefs, keep a childlike open-mindedness, and don't forget to ask the most important question of all, "Why?" You'll be surprised how many of them have no foundation at all when you ask this simple question.

Most of us have been hanging onto so many negative beliefs for so long, how could we possibly be able to realize and release all of them? Oftentimes, many of our false beliefs are tied to a singular core belief. When that belief is released, the other "hangers on" will have nothing to support them and simply fall away. These ideas can be so entrenched in our personalities that we don't even think about them anymore. It takes a very courageous person to scrutinize their value system in such an intimate way. To question one's deepest belief system is to actually challenge the "self," ego, or small (i). In other words, if my X belief isn't true, then Y isn't either, and that makes Z completely invalid. You may have a belief structure similar to this.

X: *I'm plain-looking. That's what mother always said.*

Y: *Plain-looking people are unattractive to the opposite sex.*

Z: *Because I'm unattractive, I will end up alone.*

If you release the core belief that you're plain-looking, you'll automatically see yourself as more attractive. When you feel more attractive, the idea of living your life alone just won't be believable anymore. It's these kinds of realizations that start a row of dominos falling in a chain reaction that the ego perceives as an annihilation of the false "self," or (i), and will put up somewhat of a fight to survive. If X, Y, and Z aren't true . . . then who am I? That's why you will feel some resistance at first, but make no mistake: you are the only one in control of this process.

Here's another way to look at it. Think of your belief system like a tree with thousands of branches extending outward from a single trunk. The trunk is the core belief that supports and feeds all the other beliefs. That's why it can seem difficult to remove a particular belief if we haven't eliminated the original source that's supporting it. If we cut off a branch, the tree just grows a new one. If we chop the tree down at the base, all the branches fall with it.

If we trace most of our beliefs back to their source, nearly all of us will find they're emanating from a core belief that's similar to *I'm not lovable, I don't deserve love, I'm not enough* or *There's something wrong with me.* As we think, so our lives are mirrored back to us by what we create. Yet, we never seem to make the connection between why we never have enough money, our romantic partners are never faithful, or we keep losing out on job promotions. These seemingly different problems are actually all the *same problem* when the root cause is examined.

These are examples of positive and negative core belief structures you might recognize.

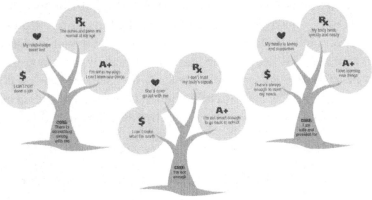

Core Belief Structure

The mistake most people make is not going deep enough. They make a sincere attempt to change their thoughts, but because they're trying to alter a surface belief and not the supporting one beneath it, little progress is made. It's like someone who's completely overwhelmed living life as a "people-pleaser," always doing things for others with no time left of their own. They can't say 'No' to other people. They might choose the new belief, "It's good to take time for myself," or "It's easy to say, No." That's a good start, except for the fact that the root thought for most people-pleasers tends to be, "I'm not enough." That's why they do so many things for other people. They feel others will only value them for what they can do for them and not for who they are. In order for change to happen, the new thought choice has to start at that level.

Change & Choice

Once we don't believe we're unattractive, lazy, hopeless, untalented, or any other lie, we can replace it with a thought that is healing. How do we do that? The same way we acquired the negative one. *We choose it.* When it comes to believing anything, the choice is yours. You get to believe it or not, and as you believe, so it is done unto you by the laws of the Universe. Buddha said, "All we are is the result of what we have thought." Christ said, "As a man thinketh, so it is done unto him."

Through our God-given free will to choose whatever we would believe and think from moment to moment, we create our lives. Within that simple principle lies complete responsibility and complete power.

The misconception in this process is that, even if you *do* expose negative core beliefs, actually changing them is difficult. Somehow these beliefs are locked away in our subconscious behind a huge steel door, where we have no access to them. We're condemned to live by their blind, driving forces. This just isn't the case. If the subconscious were completely inaccessible, we would never have been able to have exposed our hidden beliefs through the work we've done here. It's also frustrating when someone says a particular belief is "deep-seated" and difficult to access. How deeply buried can it be? The average human brain is only five-inches long and less than four-inches deep. It's really only a matter of how long you've been habitually thinking in a certain way. Yes, thinking is a habitual activity, and like any habit, it can be changed, but it takes awareness, patience, and perseverance. Even though a small stream looks like a gentle force, over time it will cut through rock.

Because your negative beliefs are stored in your subconscious, that means they are *below* or *subject to* your conscious mind. Like a child, it does not discriminate or reason. It will take any concept that's forwarded to it by the conscious mind and immediately work to bring the idea to fruition. That's why hypnotism works so well. While the conscious mind is asleep, suggestions can be offered directly to the subconscious with no resistance. In our waking lives, we have access to our subconscious by what we choose to think. Whatever idea we choose to accept and believe with conviction as true for us will be passed on to our subconscious and eventually created in our lives. Remember, if you think it's difficult to change your mind, that's a belief, too . . . and as you believe, so it is for you.

Switching Channels

When we release old beliefs and choose new ones, it's like we're switching channels on a radio or television. In fact, it's very similar to that process, because every thought has its own individual frequency vibration that resonates in our bodies when we think it. It's as if your body is a radio transmission tower sending signals out into the Universe that's returning back to you matching life circumstances. Based on what you're thinking at any given time, your body is emitting a specific, measurable bioelectrical magnetic field. Metaphysics calls this field your personal aura. Even though we can't see it, we can sense it. How many times has a stranger given you a "bad vibe," or have you met someone who has a fantastic, "magnetic" personality? That's the power of personal bioelectrical fields either attracting or repelling each other. If we look at all the bioelectrical wavelengths known, from X-rays to microwaves, it's clear that the range we can actually measure is very small. The range we actually see with our naked eyes (visible light) is the smallest of them all. The spectrum extends on into infinity, well beyond our measuring capabilities. That's where thought frequencies exist.

Electromagnetic Wave Spectrum

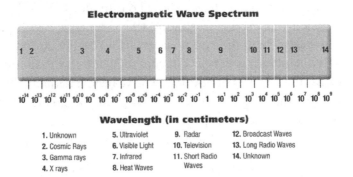

Wavelength (in centimeters)

1. Unknown	5. Ultraviolet	9. Radar	12. Broadcast Waves
2. Cosmic Rays	6. Visible Light	10. Television	13. Long Radio Waves
3. Gamma rays	7. Infrared	11. Short Radio	14. Unknown
4. X rays	8. Heat Waves	Waves	

When we switch channels on a television or radio, what do we see or hear between the old and new frequencies? Static. That's what we experience as we release old beliefs: resistance or mental static. Don't let that discourage you. It's just a part of the change process. You are literally changing the channels of your mind. The amount of static and resistance you experience depends on how far apart the frequencies are of where you're at now and where you'd like to be. There's less static between 98.1 and 98.5 on your radio dial than there is going to 107. That's why it can seem so difficult to switch from the thought pattern, *"I'm hopeless and unattractive,"* to *"I'm empowered and beautiful."* It's always best to choose a new belief that's closer to where you are at the moment. Once that idea feels secure, you can keep changing mental channels until you reach the one that serves you best. So in this case, change might begin instead by identifying attractive *qualities* about yourself, thus moving from *"I'm unattractive"* to *"My kindness appeals to others."*

THE POWER OF PATIENCE

Have patience and persistence. It doesn't matter if you're going from Los Angeles to Las Vegas by car, airplane, or on foot. There may be a big difference as to when you arrive, but one thing is **absolutely guaranteed:** As long as you stay pointed in the same direction, you **WILL** get there. The famous designer Coco Chanel was interviewed about how she created such a massive fashion empire after suffering so many setbacks. The interviewer was looking for some secret formula to success, yet her response was as simple as it was profound. She said, "I just kept going."

No one goes from A to Z in a single leap. Even an airplane experiences turbulence between altitudes, but eventually it's smooth sailing again. The idea is to continually move your thought process up to higher frequencies with the least amount of resistance. Remember, life is an inside job. All creation begins in the microcosm and is *revealed* in the macrocosm, involution to evolution. A seed is planted in the ground. The work that is done in the ground pushes a sprout out into the world. The work that is done in the sprout pushes branches out further still. The work that's done in the branches pushes outward to a bud at the end of a stem. The work done in the bud causes the rose to fold outward into its final purpose. This is the path of all creation. It will never be any other way. Financial troubles and financial success, weight gain and weight loss, are all achieved in the same way. The outside world is a world of "effects," the *end* of the creative process. The cause is always internal.

That's why diets will never work. Dieters are toiling away at the end of an assembly line wondering why their final product never changes. Be sure to give yourself credit for every step forward you take. You've embarked on a process of personal growth that 90% of the population will never take. They're constantly fighting the world "out there." It's always the fault of the ex-husband, terrible boss, low salary, bad economy, crazy drivers, or pushy family members. What they don't realize is that there is no "out there." There's only an "in here." That's all there's ever been and ever will be.

Reality Check... Believe It or Not

✓ Our thoughts arise from our beliefs.

✓ As children, we chose to accept negative beliefs about ourselves provided by our caregivers.

✓ A belief is just someone else's opinion you've adopted. That's all.

✓ We create our own reality and truth by the beliefs we choose to accept.

✓ Be like a child and challenge old beliefs by asking, *"Why?"*

✓ Releasing old beliefs is an *undoing*, a letting go that is an action of EASE.

✓ We adopt healthy beliefs the same way we acquired the old ones. We choose them.

✓ A *belief* needs to be defended. A *known* needs no explanation. It simply IS.

✓ What you *feel you deserve* will always override what you *think you want*.

✓ There is only ONE creative force in the universe. We perceive it as "good" or "bad" based on the consequences of how we're using it.

✓ The creator is not his creation. Don't be fooled by your senses!

✓ Your material world is the result of what has happened, but NOT *what's happening*.

✓ Life is always playing catch-up to your thoughts, so have patience and persistence.

✓ Choose affirmations with words that elicit a powerful emotional response for you.

Food for Thought

Family Tree

Free association is a great way to bypass your conscious mind and uncover limiting subconscious beliefs. Answer the questions below as quickly as you can, giving yourself **no time** to think or self-censor. Place those beliefs in different places in the outline below and see if you can find a common thread or core belief that links all of them. Once you've found it, you can create a new core belief with words that excite and empower you.

I am _____

My body is _____

My appearance is _____

My mother is _____

My father is _____

My family is _____

My job is _____

Men are _____

Women are _____

Money is _____

Music is _____

Sex is _____

My health is _____

I can _____

I can't _____

I should _____

I shouldn't _____

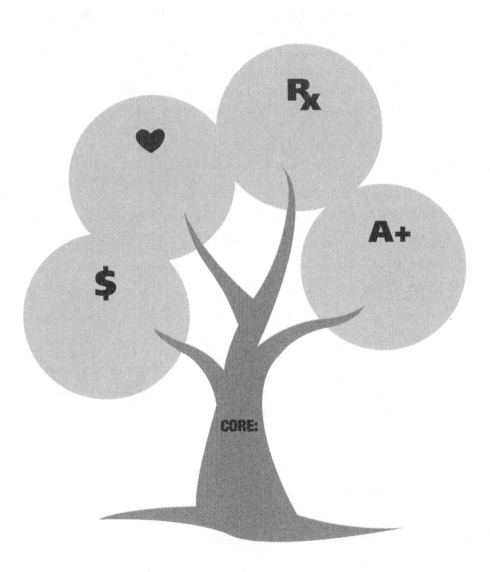

Core Belief Structure

CHAPTER 3

FEEL IT TO HEAL IT

~~~

"The subconscious does not originate ideas but accepts as true those which the conscious mind feels to be true and in a way known only to itself objectifies the accepted ideas. Therefore, through his power to imagine and feel, and his freedom to choose the idea he will entertain, man has control over creation."

—Neville Goddard, author

Learn to become conscious of how you feel in any moment. Too often, we shut our pain off because we want to avoid feeling it. Many people are anesthetized to their own feelings in this very way. Because they don't want to feel pain, they shut down emotionally. The problem with this "survival tactic" is that feelings are our "canary in the coal mine" when it comes to creating things we want in our lives. They immediately tell us what our vibration is and if we're attracting something positive or negative in every moment. If we can't feel or identify our feelings, we're creating a life by default and that's a very unsatisfying way to live.

We can't be selective about which emotions we'd like to feel. If we avoid pain and anger, that only dampens our ability to feel joy and compassion. Like black and white, summer and winter, yin and yang, our positive and negative feelings are two sides of the same coin. If you avoid painful feelings, you'll be muting your ability to experience joy, gratitude, and happiness in their fullest forms. To know what true joy is, we must have experienced true pain at some point. Otherwise, how could we identify it? We need to contrast it with something. Remember, this is a universe based on balance.

Emotions are incredibly powerful, creative forces in our lives. I like to call them e-motions or energy-in-motion. I'm sure you've felt the exhilaration of excitement fluttering through your body or the contracting waves of anger. Because our bodies are made up of moving energetic particles, humans are designed to receive an emotion, experience it fully, and then allow it to pass through us and ultimately exit. It's like someone being struck by lightning. This incredible force of energy creates a mark where it enters the body. It travels a specific route inside and then leaves an additional mark where it has exited. Some cultures practice funeral wailing to allow grief to be fully processed by the body and the excess energy expended. If we avoid our emotions, all we do is absorb the energy like a sponge. It usually becomes stored in our bodies in areas that correlate with the negative experience that generated the feeling. For instance, if someone never fully processed the pain of their relationship breakup, the energy is usually stored in the heart. Anger issues are stored in the head. Fear issues are stored in the gut, and so on. By doing this, we may buy ourselves some time, but at the ultimate cost of our health. Wherever blocked energy resides, problems exist. In the words of author, Karol Kuhn Truman, "Feelings buried alive never die."[13] We think we're being strong when we resist powerful emotions, but when strong winds blow, it's the soft reeds waving with the wind that survive. The tall rigid trees get snapped off in the midst of the force.

YOUR RESET BUTTON

Emotions are signposts that tell us if we're creating lives in a positive or negative way. For healing, it's essential to feel them, but not wallow in them. If someone makes an unkind gesture about your weight or you lose your job, it's okay and healthy to cry for an hour or even a day. If you're still crying four weeks later, that's a problem. As humans, we can do two things that no other living creature on this planet can do: laugh and cry. I believe these abilities are divine gifts. They're our spiritual reset buttons, our way of clearing our emotional palette when we're stuck in a negative energy pattern. If you're having a down moment, you know how great it can feel when a friend makes you laugh. You also know how tremendously relieving it feels when you allow yourself a good hard cry over something. In either case, you've dispelled your negative emotion and can get back to a more positive vibration.

Cluing In

Who can keep track of all their thoughts? We have thousands of thoughts in a single day. I'm sure you've had times where you're not aware of thinking anything in particular, but you're just in a bad mood, feeling out of sorts. You don't know why. You just are. Clearly, you're thinking something negative that's lowering your vibration and by universal law, drawing more negative situations to you that will match how you feel in that moment. That's why it's so important to be clued into how you're feeling, because you won't always be able to identify specifically what you're thinking some times. As long as you can identify how you feel, you can use your emotional reset buttons and change your course. Even if you don't know what you're thinking that's making you feel badly, you are, in fact, thinking something negative. Thought always precedes emotion. It never happens the other way around. Before you can feel angry, you have to think, *"That salesman ripped me off."* By staying connected to your spirit, you'll become much more aware of how and why you react to things, because there's no such thing as feeling something for no reason.

Feeling as Fuel

You see, while it's essential to understand what you're thinking, it's equally important to understand what you're feeling, because **feeling is the language of the universe**. It's estimated there are 6,909 different languages spoken on Earth[14], but when it comes to moving energy, the universe speaks only one. Feeling is the fuel that moves all energy. You'll see this demonstrated in some amazing research in the next chapter. Feeling is the fuel for your thoughts. It's what gives them the power and force to literally move matter.

Anything you feel strongly about is moving into your life much faster than something you're indifferent about. If you causally think, *"That was a great dessert. Good choice,"* that carries almost no emotional weight, and not much moves across the universal energy grid. If, however you think, *"I **never** should have had dessert. I have **no** discipline,"* your thoughts are powerfully charged with guilt and regret. The universe doesn't hear the words *dessert* or *discipline*. It's "hearing" that you feel guilty and regretful, and in that moment is working to create circumstances where you continue to feel that way, starting with stepping on the scale the next morning.

Priority One

Knowing this, we realize that we don't create our lives quite so much by what we're thinking about but by what we're **feeling** about. Understanding our thought process can help us choose better thoughts, which will result in better feelings, because—as we've already discovered—a thought always comes before a feeling. That's why it's so important that you **make feeling good your top priority** as you move throughout your day. It doesn't matter how you do it. Just do it. If it's visiting with friends, do it. If it's a walk in the park, do it. If it's playing with your pet, do it. If it's watching a funny movie, do it. As you generate the energy of good feelings, more good energy will be returned to you in the form of good things happening in your life. All the things you want, whether it's a beautiful body, great health, a better job, or a relationship are things you desire because you'll feel good by having them. Doesn't it make sense, then, that all good things are on the frequency of feeling good? So, *feel good now*, and the more powerful the emotional shift you make, the faster you'll see your life conditions begin to change.

The idea here isn't to *not* feel bad. A lot of people think not feeling bad is feeling good. No, feeling good is feeling GOOD! Not feeling bad could mean that you just feel okay or alright. If that's the case, then you'll be creating a life that's just okay or mediocre. You certainly don't want or deserve that. A clever way to keep in touch with what you're bringing into your life is to pretend you've got an invisible fairy godmother gently floating above your right shoulder all the time. She doesn't speak a word of English. The only means of communication you have with her is through your feelings. If you're happy, she assumes you want more happiness. If you're angry, she sees it as a request to get more of that. You could also see the universe as a giant copy machine: whatever you put into it will generate an exact duplicate that's returned to you.

Affirmation Overload

Feeling is extremely important when it comes to using affirmations. Used correctly, affirmations can be powerful tools for change. Unfortunately, many people use them with the best of intentions but with the reverse effect. We've already seen that repeating, *"I'm thin and beautiful,"* a thousand times will do you no good if your mind is screaming back, "NO, YOU'RE NOT." In such cases, you can actually reinforce your negative belief.

The key to affirmations isn't in the words you say or how many times you say them. It's in the **feeling** the words generate for you. When you've uncovered negative beliefs, you can create affirmations to counteract them. Even so, it's not as simple as changing the negative thought from, *"I'm fat,"* to *"I'm thin."* Those stubborn physical senses will skew your view of the truth every time you look in a mirror. Whatever affirmation you choose, it has to feel true for you NOW. Say this statement out loud: *"I'm thin, gorgeous, and full of energy."* What did you feel? Now speak this phrase: *"I'm discovering my optimal weight and vitality."* What did you feel now? You probably felt much less resistance with the second affirmation. Why? Because it includes elements that are true for you at this moment. You ARE in the process of reaching your ideal weight simply because you're reading this book. Your subconscious recognizes that fact and offers no resistance to it. That's why it's good to start affirmations with phrases such as, *"I'm discovering,"* *"I'm realizing,"* *"I'm becoming,"* and then finish them with words that generate GOOD feelings for you.

Remember, the emphasis is always on the feelings and NOT the words themselves. The universe doesn't speak English! Affirmations are only tools to generate feelings. If the feelings aren't there, your words aren't plugged into universal energy. We've all walked into any number of religious services in our lives only to see hundreds of people parroting on words in unison to prescribed prayers, completely detached from what they're saying. This is why religious texts tell us, "Do not use vain repetitions as the heathen do," if we are to see real change in our lives.

Think about it this way: Which registers more deeply with you, someone saying, "I love you," or someone embracing you? With an embrace, your being is flooded with love and words are unnecessary. You instantly KNOW you're loved. **That's because the subconscious works by association.** That's why when using affirmations, it's vital to follow them up with certain actions that corroborate the new idea with your subconscious. If you're affirming, *"I'm realizing my true beauty,"* then it's very important to follow that statement up with an action that makes you FEEL beautiful. Perhaps it's getting a makeover. There are several exercises included in this program that allow you to anchor your affirmations in your consciousness in exactly this way.

Use all the resources you can to get yourself feeling the way you want to feel. Remember, you're not feeling the way you are today because of material circumstances. You're experiencing the circumstances because of how you've been habitually feeling and thinking. Life is not happening ahead of you. It's following you. Any time you have a thought and a feeling that are in conflict, it is the feeling that will rule the day: always.

REALITY CHECK... FEEL IT TO HEAL IT

✓ If you can't feel or identify your feelings, you won't know what you're thinking . . . or creating in your life.

✓ Emotions are energy-in-motion and should pass through us by fully expressing how we feel.

✓ Emotional energy that is not fully expended becomes blocked in our bodies and creates health problems.

✓ Laughing and crying are your emotional reset buttons. Use them to throw off excess energy and return to a more healing state of mind.

✓ Thought always precedes feeling. You can't feel something without thinking something first.

✓ Feeling is the language of the universe.

✓ Affirmations have no power unless the words make you *feel* something.

✓ Feeling is the fuel that moves all energy.

✓ The universe is listening to how you feel, not to what you say.

✓ Feeling just okay or fine creates a life that is just "okay."

✓ Make feeling GOOD your **top priority** each day.

✓ Your subconscious **works by association**.

✓ Mentally anchor your affirmations with actions that *validate* them through a *physical experience*.

✓ Any time there is a conflict between a thought and a feeling, the feeling wins the day.

FOOD FOR THOUGHT

The Feeling Finder

Your ideal weight or anything else you desire in life has its own vibrational frequency. You might think you have no idea what it feels like to live in your perfect body, but that's not true. You already experience those feelings in other areas of life. The idea is to recognize when you're feeling those emotions and magnify them by doing more of those activities. The universe is listening to how you *feel* and will bring you more things to help you continue to feel that way . . . and that includes all the things you want. Use the statements below to discover how having your desires will make you feel and what you can do more of to amplify those feelings.

Example:

Weight: When I am at my ideal weight,
I will feel CONFIDENT, BEAUTIFUL and CAREFREE.

I feel confident now when *I'm teaching others* and *express my talents.*

I feel beautiful now when I *get dressed up* or *have a spa treatment.*

I feel carefree now when I *drive my convertible with the top down* and *walk in nature.*

Weight: When I'm at my ideal weight, I will feel _____

_____

_____

I feel _____ now when I _____

_____

I feel _____ now when I _____

_____

I feel _____ now when I _____

_____

Relationship: When I have my ideal relationship, I will feel _____

_____

_____

I feel _____ now when I _____

_____

I feel _____ now when I _____

_____

I feel _____ now when I _____

_____

_____

Job: When I have my ideal job, I will feel _____

_____

I feel _____ now when I _____

_____

I feel _____ now when I _____

_____

I feel _____ now when I _____

_____

CHAPTER 4

WHAT DID YOU SAY?

THE POWER OF WORDS

Be careful of your thoughts, for your thoughts become your words.
Be careful of your words, for your words become your actions.
Be careful of your actions, for your actions become your habits.
Be careful of your habits, for your habits become your character.
Be careful of your character, for your character becomes your destiny.

—Chinese Proverb

"Be careful what you say. Your tongue can be a deadly weapon.
Don't let it go off accidentally."

—Stephen D. Glass, author

"Never miss a good chance to shut up."

—Will Rogers, humorist, social commentator

We've already learned that everything in the universe is energy in different states of vibration. Therefore everything has its own frequency, like a guitar string that is plucked and creates a specific musical note. We also know that words have very powerful vibrations based on how they make us feel. This is why it's so important to not only be conscious of the words we choose when affirming our good, but to become aware of how we casually use words to sabotage ourselves.

Don't Say It

Perhaps you've had an experience like this. You're with a group of friends at an amusement park and you decide to take a ride on the Ferris wheel. When you're at the very top, gazing at the beautiful view, one of your friends decides to be a smart aleck and says, *"I wonder what would happen if the bolt holding our car broke right now."* Terrified, your immediate response is, *"Don't say it!"* Even though you may not have really believed your cart would break loose and plunge to the ground, you instinctively responded the way you did because, subconsciously, **you know the power of words**. Every word we read, speak, or write has the power to change our personal energy vibration and ultimately bring its reality into existence.

Words are one of our greatest tools when choosing to change our lives. It's astonishing, then when we realize how often we use words to unconsciously undo our best efforts. Some of the most damaging words are the ones we don't say, at least not out loud. It's our self-talk, the conversation we have with ourselves inside our heads when we fall off another diet wagon. We say to ourselves, *"I have no discipline. I'm so lazy. I deserve to be fat."* At work we might say, *"I blew that presentation. I knew I'd screw it up. Now I'll never get the promotion."*

These kinds of internal interactions create a very strong energetic imprint on our bodies and on the outward conditions of our lives. It does absolutely no good to affirm something positive for yourself outwardly if this kind of emotional tug-of-war is happening on the inside. It's important in these situations to be kind to ourselves, to give ourselves the permission to make mistakes. Why would we judge ourselves by a standard up to which we'd never hold anyone else? In these moments, it's best to take a step back and **release your judgment**. When there's no judgment, there is no "good" or "bad" valuation put on something. When you view the situation from an emotional distance, you can see it for what it is. A decision was made. That decision created a specific result. So, you make a *new* decision. It's only when we extract the emotional charge from situations like this that we can have the clarity to consciously direct our lives. Otherwise, you create a false self or (i) that's defined by its circumstances. Non-judgment is a foundational element in all spiritual practice. The mystics and sages of old knew this and have always taught that we should not judge our fellow man. They also knew that, like love, you cannot provide non-judgment to others if you are unable to offer it to yourself first.

The Internal Parent

We tend to treat ourselves the way we've been treated in the past, mostly by our parents. It again goes back to the power of habit and our conscious re-creating what we perceive as "normal" for us. It's a process known as Self-Parenting in psychology circles. If you can, stop in the middle of a self-talk rant and take note of specific words or phrases you use. Chances are, they're the same names, words, or phrases your parents used in moments of unkindness. You'll see that it's not really you doing the talking. It's just the play button being pushed on an old tape recorder that's blaring someone else's outdated negative beliefs.

The idea behind Self-Parenting is to "re-parent" the innocent, childlike spirit that's inside your heart with the compassion, patience, and love it never received. When we become aware of negative self-talk rants, then we can interrupt them with a more supportive dialogue. When I say dialogue, I mean exactly that. Have a real conversation with your child spirit, your true essence that's pure, does its best, and always acts out of the most loving intentions. In the midst of a guilt trip over having too much dessert, you might say to your inner child, *"It's okay. I understand. I love chocolate, too. I know how yummy it is and you should have it, just maybe not so much. If we have too much too often, then it's not special anymore, and I want it to be a special treat for you because you deserve it. So, maybe we'll have it again in a couple of days."*

Don't try to intellectualize with the innocent, childlike part of yourself. Use simple, comforting words and speak exactly as if you were speaking to a child. You'll be surprised how quickly these kind, nurturing words can dissolve critical self-talk and their negative emotions. It also helps if you can speak the dialogue out loud. If it stays in your head, it's just an intellectual exercise. When you speak it out loud, it becomes active and you're experiencing it with your own senses. Every cell of your body is listening to every word you speak, and the most precious, healing, intimate sound it will ever hear is the sound of its own voice.

Perfectly Imperfect

Most negative self-talk happens when we fail to live up to self-imposed, ridiculously high standards that no one else could possibly achieve. When we grow up in an environment that's dysfunctional or imperfect, we assume that there's something wrong with us, and that if we can somehow do it *right*, *better*, or *perfectly*, then the situation will be better, too. As a result, we go through life treating ourselves with such rigidity and perfectionism that it becomes impossible to make a mistake. Inevitably, we *will* make mistakes, but we won't allow ourselves to receive the lessons they offer because we're too busy yelling at ourselves. When we deny ourselves the chance to make mistakes, we deny ourselves half of our learning opportunities in life. We learn half of what we need from our success and the other half from our failures. What we learn from our most recent failure only leads to the next success. Thomas Edison failed 1,000 times before he was successful in creating the light bulb. He would later say that he didn't fail 1,000 times. Inventing the light bulb had 1,000 steps. Interesting perspective.

Knowing what doesn't work is just as important as knowing what does. Mistakes are good. They point us in a whole new direction. How many walls will a mouse run into before he finally exits a maze? If it weren't for the roadblocks, he would never have found the way out. Perfectionism holds us back. It makes us apprehensive and afraid to take chances because it might not turn out the way we want it to. Ultimately, our life becomes stuck and we don't move forward. A life lived in fear really is a life half-lived. The Rev. Robert Schuller said it best when he said, "It's better to do something imperfectly than nothing perfectly." NBA superstar Michael Jordan also knew the perfection of being imperfect when he said, "You miss 100% of the shots you don't take."

THE BODY ELECTRIC

The human body is a network of bioelectromagnetic energy constantly interacting with the infinite field of energy in which it exists. We know that energy is highly influenced by our thoughts. We also know that the human body is 60% water, with 2/3 of that amount being intracellular, or existing inside our cells.[15] Water is highly conductive to electricity when it contains charged particles, like the trace minerals we have in our bodies. When we look at the fact that human beings are mostly water combined with a highly conductive agent, it's clear that our bodies were designed as the optimal machine to transfer and process electromagnetic energy.

This is why the words we speak, write, and listen to have such an immediate impact on us. Their positive or negative vibrations create a ripple effect across this internal ocean, accelerated by the conducting agents and delivered to every single cell of our bodies in a fraction of a second, millions of times a day. Getting into the habit of only speaking and thinking good things about yourself and others is far more than just positive thinking. It's a matter of life and death.

WORDS & WATER

Nowhere has the impact of the energetics of words been more vividly displayed than in the work of internationally renowned researcher and author Masaru Emoto. He had been working as an alternative healthcare physician and healer in Japan in the 1990s. He instinctively knew about the transformative relationship between energy and water based on the results he'd been experiencing with his patients. Even so, he had no way to demonstrate this profound effect to others. People so often believe only what they can see. Eventually, Emoto developed a high-definition, high-speed form of photography that could capture the image of water the moment it began to freeze and form ice crystals.

Water that has been polluted or contains additives such as chlorine and fluoride, like all tap water, will not form crystals as it freezes. The additives alter its structure, rending it impure and prevent this natural process. When frozen, water that is pure and free of unnatural ingredients will form the most intricate, balanced, luminescent crystals resembling snowflakes.

In his initial experiments, Emoto photographed frozen tap water samples from Tokyo, which is often held as some of the worst municipal water in the world. The photos showed dark brown and gray misshapen blobs similar to an oil slick. The water was incapable of crystallizing. Later, he photographed a sample of the same water that he'd kept in a small vial on his desk with a label reading "LOVE" attached to the outside. This sample, of the exact same water which received no purification treatment, formed perfectly-shaped, radiantly white, symmetrical ice crystals. The difference was astonishing. Some samples even took on the physical attributes of the word they were exposed to, as if to communicate symbolically that it understood even the context of the word. A sample exposed to the words "WEDDED LOVE" showed two perfect ice crystals entwined within each other, almost like married partners. Another specimen labeled "FAMILY LOVE" revealed three layers of crystals nesting together to possibly symbolize three generations: grandparents, parents, and children, or perhaps husband, wife, and child. As Emoto continued, his experiments showed that water exposed to any positive words such as "PEACE," "RESPECT," and "THANK YOU" always formed beautiful crystals, while samples exposed to words such as "HATE" and "I WILL KILL YOU" were incapable of doing so.

As the Part, So the Whole

To further demonstrate this phenomenon, Emoto gathered a small band of volunteers to gather at a lakeside in Carapicuiba, Brazil, where the water had been polluted by industrialization. The volunteers held hands in a circle around a small sample of the lake water. After a short period of sending loving intentions toward the sample, the water could form beautiful crystals. It would be discovered later as an astonishing surprise that not only did the structure of the water in the sample jar change, but the water in the entire lake, as well. Samples taken from the lake were forming perfectly symmetrical crystals once more as if to communicate the spiritual axiom, *As is the part, so is the whole.*

Emoto's research not only demonstrated the power of our thought-based and written words but our spoken language, as well. To do so, he placed cooked rice samples in two jars. He used cooked rice because of the water content. One sample was labeled, "Thank You." The other was labeled, "You Fool." The samples were left in an elementary school classroom where the children were instructed to speak the words on the labels to each jar for 30 seconds twice a day. At the end of 30 days, the rice labeled "Thank You" had not changed or begun to decompose. It looked like it did the day it was put in the jar, while the other sample had shriveled into a black mass. Many others have re-created this same experiment, some with samples up to 1½ years old. I highly recommend viewing Emoto's crystal and rice samples in his series of books, *The Hidden Messages in Water*.[16] The visible power of words in any form has never been more impressively displayed.

The Last Laugh

Maintaining a positive and nurturing inner dialogue is a challenge for anyone. For those struggling with weight, however, it's what they choose to say externally that gives away the war of words on the inside. Too often, they make themselves the butt of their own jokes in social situations. They assume that if they're the ones to turn their weight problems into punch lines first, anything anyone else might say won't sting as badly because they will have had the last laugh. They will have exercised a certain amount of control over the situation.

The problem with self-deprecation is that universal energy doesn't have a sense of humor. It hears the intention behind and acts upon every single word we speak. Someone might be laughing when they step into a swimming pool and say, *"Look out now, here comes the tidal wave!"* Others might laugh at the joke, but the subtle energy inside the body can't be fooled. It hears the entire subtext. *"I'm so embarrassed. I look hideous in this bathing suit. I don't deserve to be here, so I'll make a joke and apologize for my existence."*

In these situations, some age-old advice from our mothers becomes very valuable. If you can't say anything nice (about yourself), don't say anything at all. In most cases, self-deprecation backfires. Almost no one is paying attention to your weight in social situations. They're too busy doing their own thing until you bring attention to it. The very thing you don't want (everyone fixated on your weight), you actually create by making a joke out of it. In addition, you attract more negative energy and situations to you by the words and intentions you're using. Remember that words have incredible power, and every cell of your body is listening.

Reality Check...
What Did You Say? The Power of Words

✓ Every word has a specific positive or negative vibration based on your emotion attached to it.

✓ The power of words is the same whether they're written, spoken, or unspoken.

✓ Some of the most powerful words we use are in our mental self-talk.

✓ Using non-judgment allows us to learn from our mistakes and neutralize negative self-talk.

✓ The way we habitually treat ourselves in self-talk is reminiscent of how we were treated as children by the adults in our lives.

✓ Negative self-talk usually involves unrealistic standards of perfectionism.

✓ Failure is a necessary step toward success. Negative self-talk keeps us from learning the lesson and moving forward.

✓ The water in our cells actually conducts the energy from the words we use, like electricity.

✓ Beware of self-deprecation. The universe has no sense of humor!

FOOD FOR THOUGHT

Negating Negatives

I've said this program is NOT a diet. It's not even close. While you're participating in this program however, I'd like to you go on a diet of negatives. That means from the day you begin until the day you end (and hopefully beyond) you eliminate using negative words of any kind. Try eliminating the words *no, not, can't, won't, don't, couldn't, wouldn't, shouldn't,* and so on. Instead of saying, "*I don't want to go out tonight,*" say, "*I'd rather stay in.*" Instead of "*I couldn't wait any longer,*" say, "*I had to go.*" This is tricky at first, but you'll get the hang of it. You'll be surprised how soon you'll be able to catch yourself and choose different words. By reducing our use of negative terms, we automatically begin to think with a positive slant. We even feel better and start to attract positive things. This exercise is very simple, but also very powerful.

I'd also like you to abolish the word "should" from your vocabulary. It doesn't matter how it's used, it always implies a level of judgment which breeds fear, guilt, and shame as by-products. If you "should" be doing something and you're not, it implies that you're acting irresponsibly or wasting time. Replace it with "could." It means you have choices. It gives you power, not an ultimatum. So instead of saying, "*I should be studying instead of going out to dinner,*" you can say, "*I could study beforehand and maybe an hour afterward.*" Making this choice is a small but effective way to treat your childlike spirit with kindness. It's also a good stress reliever. Give yourself a break and stop should-ing all over the place!

Upgrade / Downgrade

Because words can generate powerful responses, it's beneficial to capitalize on their emotional impact. When we speak with awareness, we have power over our words. They do not have power over us. Bumping up the intensity of your positive word choices can really lift your personal energy, while downplaying the negatives can keep them from dragging you down. For example: If someone asks, "*How are you?*" you might respond, "*Fine.*" If so, you're creating a day and a life that's just "fine." Try upgrading that response to *good, great, fantastic, terrific, wonderful,* or any other choice that lifts your personal energy vibration. In contrast, instead of calling something "*infuriating,*" you might downgrade your word choice to *irritating, troublesome,* or *annoying.* See how many times you can keep upgrading the positive terms and downgrading the negative terms on the next page.

Ugly   Striking   Eccentric   Unique

Failure _____

Terrible _____

Depressed _____

Angry _____

Cool   Clever   Amazing   Ingenious

Funny _____

Pretty _____

Smart _____

CHAPTER 5

CONSCIOUSNESS IS KING

〰

*"No problem can be solved from the same level
of consciousness that created it."*

—Albert Einstein, physicist

*"Man, through the medium of a controlled waking dream
can determine his future."*

—Neville Goddard, author

"Know ye not, ye are gods."

—Hermetic aphorism

Changing our lives for the better means becoming fully conscious, but conscious of what and how? What exactly *is* consciousness, anyway? The term *consciousness* is tossed around quite a bit in self-help, metaphysical, and even scientific circles. It's become a pop-culture buzzword that everyone's "into" but few seem to really understand. It can create confusion and even seem intimidating. When we hear someone speak of consciousness, it's usually a New Age guru or respected spiritual leader who can leave us with the impression that it's an achievement beyond the "average person." Somehow, the only way to attain true consciousness is to forsake all worldly possessions, retreat to an ancient temple in the Far East, and pray for 12 hours a day. That's not true, but it is how we end up feeling because there's so much confusion surrounding the idea of consciousness. The truth is that consciousness, like the rest of life, is simple. It's so simple that you don't have to go anywhere to find consciousness. It's right where you are because it's *what you are.*

GHOST IN THE MACHINE

Dr. Wilder Penfield was a world-renowned neurosurgeon who pioneered the study of right brain / left brain theory and developed treatments for patients with severe epilepsy in the first half of the 20th Century. He spent most of his career attempting to establish a scientific basis for the existence of the human soul. His experiments included stimulating the part of a patient's brain that would make the right arm rise involuntarily. When asked if he or she was assisting the process in any way, the patient would respond that they were making no effort to raise the arm, yet it was. Penfield recorded the area in the brain that controlled this movement. Moments later, the doctor asked the patient to actively move their arm back down to the starting position. At that point, the patient could consciously override the process and return their arm to their side.

Penfield noted that the brain could be stimulated to move the patient's arm involuntarily. Through this exercise, he could locate *the part of the brain* that controls the motor function of movement. What he could *not* find was the place or location where *the choice* was made to lower the arm back down. He could only document the physical part of the brain that was activated *after a choice was made*, but where was the choice itself made, and by whom? No matter how sophisticated science gets, we will never be able to find the place where that choice is made, because it doesn't exist in the brain. The brain is only a tool that we choose to use as the needs calls, like an arm or leg. The entity actually making the "choice" exists outside the body in a much larger field called consciousness.

IT'S ALREADY DONE

That field includes every possible outcome to every situation you could ever imagine. Which outcomes and objects eventually manifest in our lives depend on where we focus our attention in that energy field. Because every single outcome has its own frequency, and the universe contains an infinite expanse of frequencies, we can tune into any one of them. This gives us an endless number of ways in which we can solve our problems. In fact, science tells us that these possibilities already exist. Whatever you desire—your ideal weight, life partner, health, or career—already exists because its frequency exists. If you can feel it through your imagination, you can bring it into being. It's already done. Your job is to become conscious of that frequency so its material form can be downloaded into your life. Werner Heisenberg, the Nobel Prize-winning physicist, said that we live in a "world of potentialities or possibilities rather than one of material things." It's the same reason all ancient spiritual traditions tell us that all we seek is finished even before we ask. British poet Alfred Lord Tennyson explained our personal power as being "closer than breathing and nearer than hands and feet."

THE POWER OF BEING

If the answers to our greatest needs are that close to us, it implies the solution is not in the outer world where we're so tempted to "do" this, "go" there, and "get" that to stomp out our problems. It points to something much more intimate. The solution isn't "out there." It isn't even inside of you. It's closer than that. The solution to your problem doesn't need to be found because you *are* the solution.

You become what you *are*. In his legendary work, *As a Man Thinketh*, author James Allen says, "Men do not attract that which they want, but that which they are."[17] We become in form what we are in consciousness. If consciousness isn't a function of our brains, isn't intellectual intelligence, or even our memories, then what is it? **Consciousness is beingness**. How or whatever you are "being" at this moment is what you are conscious of. If you are sad, depressed, and lonely, then that is what you are conscious of. Beingness and consciousness go hand in hand. You cannot BE sad but conscious of happiness at the same time. BEING CONSCIOUS of something is a state of KNOWING something, being in the midst of it, experiencing it NOW. We've learned that *knowing*, as opposed to believing, only comes from direct physical or emotional experience. So, to become conscious of anything, we must generate an *experience* for ourselves that allows us to *know* what it's like to be, do, or have whatever it is we desire. Remember, the subconscious creates what it *knows*, what it is aware of. To raise our level of awareness, we must raise our level of beingness. Flipping through a travel magazine and looking at the white sand and turquoise waters of the South Pacific doesn't make you conscious of it. Feeling the warmth of the sun caress your back, the tickle of the sand between your toes, and hearing the rush of ocean waves is what it means to be fully conscious of being on the beach.

This is the problem so many people have when they create "vision boards" to attract something into their lives. They may cut out photos of famous actresses and models who have the type of body they want and pin them to a bulletin board where they'll see them regularly. The problem with this approach is that just looking at the photos doesn't generate any kind of real experience. It doesn't register in the cells of their body. It doesn't tell them, *"Oh! This is what I'm supposed to be."* It's trying to work the creative process from the opposite direction; trying to make an evolution create an involution, and we already know it does NOT work that way. The involution always precedes the evolution: the microcosm to the macrocosm. Think about it. If just staring at something all day could make it manifest, then everyone who worked in a bank would be a millionaire!

BEING VS. DOING

Being is the key to conscious creation. We are called human BEINGS, not human DOINGS. Yet, we get caught up in thinking that we must HAVE something before we can DO something so we can BE something. We think that we must *have* the ideal weight before we can *do* the things we want to do (vacation, go dancing, dating, high school reunion) and then we'll *be* happy. The creative process, however, works in the opposite direction. When we're already *being* or living in the

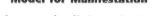

Model for Manifestation

mental state of what we want, it organically leads us to *do* all the right things to *have* our desire in the shortest amount of time, because we're acting from a place where we already ARE that which we seek. At that place, we're ONE with our dreams. *A Course in Miracles* tells us that there is no difference between being it and having it.[18] Having is a natural by-product of being.

When we come from any other level of consciousness, we're just grasping in the dark. That's why diets will always fail. You can't act from the consciousness of an overweight person who's *trying* to be a thin person. That breeds the consciousness of frustration and desperation and the universe will answer that call with more of the same.

Growth vs. Goals

When we are BEING something, our lives are growth-oriented. We understand how to raise our consciousness to reach our desires. Everything becomes an opportunity to learn how to be or *not* to be. From this place, every experience we have **is positive** because it's either telling us that the changes we're making are working or they're not. Even what's not working gives us valuable information to make the necessary changes, so it's still positive. Our desires aren't deadlines we must reach, but tools we use to raise our awareness about how life really works as we learn how to reach them.

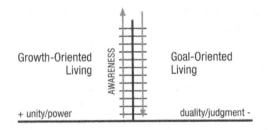

Growth-Oriented Living — AWARENESS — Goal-Oriented Living

+ unity/power — duality/judgment -

Growth/Goal Life Perspective

When we jump into DOING, our lives become goal-oriented. We become rushed and stressed out as we put timelines on everything and try to multitask our way to happiness. We become dependent on the outcome of circumstances and forced into a judgmental frame of mind. If what we're doing is working, that's "good"; if not, it's "bad." We live in a world of duality and negative interpretations. In a world of duality, there is always an opposing force, something we feel we must fight against: fight the fat, fight obesity, fight calories, etc., and wherever we apply force, we'll always get an equal amount of counterforce. It's a recipe for going nowhere.

Detachment Made Easy

It doesn't matter what we want, whether it's our ideal weight, perfect partner, radiant health, or dream home. We only want what we want for one reason: how it will make us *feel*. It's not so much about fitting into that "little black dress" as it is the feeling of freedom and sexiness you experience after slipping into it. BEING helps foster detachment from our desires. When we're BEING, we're released from angst-ridden expectations for a specific outcome because we're *already feeling* the way we'd feel if we had our desire right now. In this state of reduced resistance, our desire manifests effortlessly of its own accord and in the perfect time.

When we're BEING, we're not task-driven. We don't *have to do* things like count calories and measure food items. Our choices and actions flow spontaneously from a higher consciousness where we don't have to think about them constantly. The DOING just comes naturally.

YOUR ROLE

This doesn't mean you do nothing to obtain your desires. It just means that you **create the consciousness of having your desire first**, and then listen intuitively for what you need to do. Remember what your role is in the universal creative process. It's your responsibility to create a state of consciousness, NOT the condition. You are to create the attitude of having your desire, NOT the outcome. The end results are the work of the creative process. So BE it now. You'll be led to what you need to DO, and soon you will HAVE your desire.

This very concept appears in nearly all sacred texts. *To him that hath, it is given. To him that hath not, it is not given.* Too many people are repeating "skinny affirmations" while acting like an overweight person. That's why their affirmations don't work. Author and teacher Marianne Williamson explained it best when she said, "It's easier to act your way into a new way of thinking than it is to think your way into a new way of acting."

So act like a thin person NOW. BE a thin person NOW. Order food at a restaurant like a thin person. Eat dessert like a thin person. Walk like a thin person. Exercise like a thin person. Say, "No, thank you," to desserts like a thin person, and soon, you will be a thin person. Your body will respond and rise up to match your level of consciousness. In his legendary work, *Feeling IS the Secret*, Neville Goddard tells us that, "As you capture the feeling of the state sought, you are relieved of all effort to make it so because it already IS so."[19] Unity minister Eric Butterworth tells us that we are to "think *from* the idea and not *of* it." If we simply think of what we want, we're removed from the experience. It's like we're watching someone else in a movie. We have to generate the feelings of having what we want NOW.

A fascinating example of achieving desires through BEING comes from Archibald Alexander Leach. Born in 1904, Leach lived with an abusive, alcoholic father who eventually abandoned him and his mother. At age ten, he came home one day to find his mother missing. Relatives told him she'd gone on a long vacation and died of a heart attack while away. It wasn't until he was 31 that he would discover she was alive and had been committed to a mental institution for the last 20 years. In the midst of this seemingly insurmountable misery, he made a decision to act AS IF he already was the person he wanted to be, living the life he truly desired. His life eventually evolved to match his consciousness. Today, we know that man as legendary actor Cary Grant. He would later admit he created the Cary Grant "character" in his daily life. Commenting on his ultimate success, he said, "I pretended to be somebody I wanted to be and I finally became that person, or he became me."[20] [21] It's as Shakespeare said when he wrote, "Assume a virtue, if you have it not."

PRAYER & POWER

Our religious and spiritual traditions tell us to "pray without ceasing," but what does that mean? We can't realistically recite prayers or affirmations all day, every day until we receive an answer. It means that we are to assume the state of BEING that corresponds to our desire. The BEINGNESS or consciousness *is the prayer*: the vibrational message we're sending out into the universe to have returned to us in material form. When we're BEING in this way, we're praying 24/7. Saying traditional prayers over and over does not move the hand of the universe. If you're speaking, you're just reciting. If you're *BEING*, you're praying. Inspirational author Wallace Wattles cleverly said, "The answer to prayer is not according to your faith while you are talking, but according to your faith while you are working."[22]

BACK IN TIME

The power of your consciousness is limitless. It can even turn back time. In 1981, Harvard University psychology professor Ellen J. Langer, Ph.D. conducted one of the most dramatic research projects on the power of the mind; it still has scientists and spiritualists buzzing today. She gathered two groups of men in their seventies and eighties and took them to a secluded monastery in the Boston area two weeks apart from each other. Inside the monastery, she re-created an entire world from the 1950s. She had pink Cadillacs and Bel Airs parked outside. Walter Cronkite was on the television reporting news and reruns of *I Love Lucy* and *Leave It to Beaver* looped over and over. Copies of *LIFE Magazine* were everywhere, and all the radio broadcasts included baseball games with Mickey Mantle and music from Elvis and Buddy Holly. It was a life-size, sensory-intensive time warp.

Her original intention was to examine how pre-determined beliefs about aging affect humans physiologically. The results she found were highly unexpected and stunned everyone. The first group to enter the monastery was simply told to reminisce the good old days and have fun. The second group was told not to reminisce, but to *behave as if* they were still in the 1950s. They were instructed to completely immerse themselves in the environment and act as though they were their younger selves at that time.

At the end of just one week, the group of men who were reminiscing the past, showed improvements in all their biomarkers. Their sight, hearing, systolic blood pressure, skin elasticity, and flexibility had all improved. Their posture was better, bones stronger, and even their hands were less gnarled by arthritis. The group that was BEING in the 1950s showed *significantly* more improvement in all these areas. Even their wrinkles had faded. The evidence was showing that the aging process didn't just stop—it reversed itself! In fact, the subjects who were acting like younger men ended the experiment with bodies that, based on scientific indicators, actually *were* younger.[23] With regard to her landmark study, Dr. Langer has said, "Wherever you put your mind, the body will follow."

THE COMPANY YOU KEEP

Our environment has an enormous impact on our state of consciousness, or BEING. A significant part of that influence includes other people. I'm sure you've felt whether someone gives off a good or bad vibe when you're in their company. You're feeling their personal energy that's emanating from their current state of consciousness. As universal principle commands, energy is always drawn to energy of a similar nature. The old saying, "Birds of a feather flock together" is based in science. Someone who is cynical and loves to complain will inevitably find their way into the company of other complainers. Someone who is upbeat will gravitate toward a more positive crowd. This is the reason all groups are drawn together. They share a common consciousness that comes from relatable experiences. This is why even in larger cities, ethnic, religious and various social groups tend to pool together into specific neighborhoods.

Because we are powerfully affected by the consciousness of others, it's extremely important that we keep company with other people who uplift and support us, make us laugh and feel good. We should minimize the amount of time we spend with people who do not make us feel this way and avoid them all together, if we can.

With this in mind, I'd like to mention how support groups can be a positive or negative influence on us when we're trying to change our lives. Everyone needs support when working through life's changes. These groups can be a great tool if they help us move *forward* toward real solutions and healing. They can be a counter-productive force for us if they turn out to be a group of people getting together to commiserate over their mutual problems. This isn't to imply that they do not want to change their lives. Their intentions are sincere; however, some of these groups get quite lost in confusing their identity with their circumstance. Members can get labeled as "addicts for life" that will "always be in recovery."

Once we perceive ourselves this way, we certainly will never recover because that is what we believe and as we believe, so it is done. I see this a lot when people refer to their conditions as *my* cancer or *my* food addiction. People often identify themselves as a cancer survivor long after they've entered remission. Why on Earth would anyone consciously continue to equate themselves with cancer in the same sentence, even after the fact? To do so is to include it in your consciousness. Forget about being a cancer survivor and just be *a survivor*. We're all survivors. Anyone who wakes up tomorrow morning and draws breath is a survivor!

There is a difference between saying, "I AM a food addict," or "I AM a cancer patient," and "I have a food addiction," or "I have cancer." Having something is not BEING something. Once we incorporate a problem into our identity, the small (i) of our ego will not easily give it up. It becomes what it "is," who you "are," and it will fight tooth-and-nail to hold onto it.

When choosing a support group, use your intuition and listen to what the energy of a group is telling you. A negative person's energy is powerful enough but the energy of 15 negative people is 15 times stronger. The energetic pull of a group, for good or ill, is very powerful. That's why "mob mentality" can sweep an otherwise level-headed person away into doing things they normally wouldn't do. Cults work the same way. Always make sure that any support group you attend is focused forward toward healing and never self-identifies with the problem.

MODELS & MENTORS

Ideally, the level of consciousness you want to surround yourself with is that of someone who's already where you want to be. They're not in the midst of the problem. They've come through it and are now exuding the higher consciousness of having done so. This is an age-old practice of some of the world's richest men and women. Many of the wealthy industrialists of the last two centuries weren't born into their money. They wanted to create wealth, so they put themselves in the company of tycoons and businessmen who had the appropriate financial knowledge but also emanated a wealthy "state of mind." Many even offered to be interns, free of charge, just to be in the presence of the level of consciousness they desired. As a result, they too became multi-millionaires.

How much sense does it make to seek out a piano teacher if you want to play the trombone? If you wanted to invest some money would you take the advice of someone who's living paycheck-to-paycheck? Finding support is good. Finding a mentor is better. Does it make sense to get weight loss advice from someone who is beginning their 20th year of dieting? Maybe it's better to receive it from someone who's kept their weight off for 20 years and is now a personal trainer. Many people who have lost weight permanently did it by interviewing people who were in the place they wanted to BE now. They even interviewed people who never had an issue with food to find a model for the behavior they wanted to emulate. When we work closely with a great mentor, we become partners is progress, not commiseraters in unconsciousness.

THE TIME IS NOW

BEING something means assuming the state of it NOW. You can't BE something in the past because the past is gone. You can't BE something in the future because it isn't here, yet and when it does arrive, it will be NOW. You can only BE something NOW because NOW is all there is. Time, as we know it does not exist. It's really just an eternal procession of NOWs. That's why it's so important to BE what you want NOW because it can only happen NOW, and the future never arrives because it doesn't really exist. Albert Einstein described time as "a stubbornly persistent illusion that we help create."

Think about it. When you celebrated your 10th birthday, when did that happen? It happened in a NOW moment. When you were going to your senior prom, when did that happen? It happened in a NOW moment. When you step into that perfect outfit you've been waiting to wear and it fits perfectly, when will that happen? It will happen in a NOW moment. You put the manifestation of your dreams on hyper-speed when you adopt the consciousness of BEING what you want NOW. Being in the NOW releases us from all stress, because guilt and regret live in the artificial "past" and fear is in the "pretend" future. The only way to be truly free is to live by the words of the great philosopher and author Ram Dass, who coined the popular phrase, "BE HERE NOW." Shakespeare also shared this idea when he wrote in *Hamlet*, "Lord, we know what we are but know not what we may be." When we can learn to live our "future" desire in the NOW, magic will happen and new, liberating possibilities will start coming our way.

Reality Check... Consciousness Is King

✓ Your consciousness is your current state of BEING. It is what you *are*.

✓ To be conscious of something is to KNOW it, to experience it NOW.

✓ You can remember something from the past but you cannot BE conscious of it because consciousness is a NOW experience.

✓ Consciousness comes from a direct physical or emotional experience that allows us to KNOW what it is like to be, do or have whatever we want NOW.

✓ The universe contains the frequency of the solution to every problem. Your consciousness must match this frequency to bring it into BEING.

✓ We are human BEINGS, not human doings.

✓ BEINGNESS is a growth-centered life where situations become opportunities to learn and expand.

✓ Doing-ness is a goal-oriented life that makes our joy dependent on outcomes. It creates judgment. It locks us into a world of duality, of "good" and "bad."

✓ BEINGNESS fosters detachment because it gives us the feelings of having our desires NOW. It reduces resistance and frees us from the circumstances of outcomes.

✓ You create the consciousness of your desire, not the condition. You create the attitude, not the outcome.

✓ To pray without ceasing is to live every day in the BEINGNESS of your desire.

✓ Where your mind goes, energy flows.

✓ Never self-identify with a problem. You *have* a problem, but you are not the problem itself.

✓ Mentors are powerful influences on our consciousness.

✓ Time is an illusion. The only time anything happens is NOW.

FOOD FOR THOUGHT

Snap Out of It

Racing thoughts can whisk us right out of a "now" moment and carry us off on an obsessive internal rant. When we're not in the "now," we're not consciously creating the life we desire. If a tidal wave of negative thoughts is sweeping over you, the best way to interrupt the process is to get out of your mind. You can do that by going into your body. When our consciousness goes to the body, we become fully present in the moment. If you find that you're berating yourself with negative thoughts and can't stop them, do anything to create a physical sensation; stomp your feet on the floor, run your hands under cold water, even sing or yell out loud if you're in the car. The idea is to pull you out of your mind by engaging your physical body. At that point, you can consciously choose your next thought. I've even heard of people who wear a rubber band around their wrist and pull it now and then to snap themselves out of it.

Starring Role

From beliefs to thoughts and ultimately BEINGNESS, we create our lives from moment to moment. We're like the writer, director, and actor in our own real-life movie. Living in the state of BEING your desire now, *feeling the wish fulfilled* is the key to a true creative life. Reaching your ideal weight can create a lot of new feelings like confidence, sexiness, good humor, light-heartedness, and assertiveness. It can be tough to assume this state of BEING, especially if you've never felt any of these things before. You need a frame of reference. It's like trying to describe the color blue. You can't. You simply have to experience seeing it, and then you know what it is.

One of the best ways to find this feeling place is to think of a famous actor or actress who you admire for their personality, accomplishments, or even their great body. Study the way they move, how they carry themselves, the inflection of their voice, their sense of humor, and general disposition. As you go about your day, choose specific moments where you can assume the "role" of this person. Think of yourself AS that person in an interaction with a valet, a cashier, or a neighbor, and see how you begin to assume that state of BEING. Start slowly and work up to sustaining it in as many interactions and for as long as you can. It's not about doing an impersonation. It's about taking on the right disposition. Soon, you won't need to think of the celebrity anymore, because it will already have become your natural state of BEING.

CHAPTER 6

GOODBYE TO YOU
LETTING GO OF YOUR STORY

~~~

*"Though no one can go back and make a brand new start,
anyone can start from now and make a brand new beginning."*

—**Carl Bard**, *author*

*"There will come a time when you think everything is finished.
That will be the beginning."*

—**Louis L'Amour**, *author*

*"When I let go of what I am, I become what I might be.
When I let go of what I have, I receive what I need."*

—**Lao Tzu**, *Tao Te Ching*

There's one in every family, in every workplace, and in every social situation. You can't miss them because they're the ones who talk the loudest . . . and the longest. All you have to do is ask the forbidden question, *"How are you?"* and out will pour an endless stream of woe, tragedy, and misfortune. They may sound quite sad, but make no mistake. They love it. They love giving you all the gory details about their latest physical ailment, financial loss, or relationship disaster. They love it because they've been rehearsing it (and reliving it) for years. Telling you all their trials and tribulations confirms for them how noble they are to have suffered such injustices. If they could have done better, they would have done better if it just weren't for those nasty old fates dealing them such a rotten, unlucky hand in life.

I hardly think so.

Most of us have a string of experiences (birthplace, college years, a bad relationship, a good relationship, children, etc.) that we call our life. Whether good, bad, or a mixture of both, this "story" is how most people define themselves. It gives them a place, an identity in the world. Because of it, they stand "for" or "against" something, have been through something, accomplished something, or lost something that, for them, defines their character, their very being. This "story" is not who you are. It's simply a sequence of experiences you've created based on your beliefs and thoughts at different moments.

One of the biggest hurdles people face in healing their lives is getting stuck in the past, clinging to their story. As we've learned, time as we once thought of it, doesn't really exist. If time doesn't exist, then the past is just an illusion. In a now-centered universe, it's impossible to relive something from the past because it's dead. It's gone. It has no life force anymore. If you're bothered by something from the past, it's not the boss who fired you or the spouse who left you that's holding you back. It's your perception of the experience that's connected to a powerful belief that you keep replaying over and over that's in your way. The situation and person involved never had any power to begin with, because it's impossible for anyone else to choose your thoughts about them. So, the only person or thing that has ever been holding you back is you.

MISERY ADDICTION

Remember, this is a universe based on order. There is no such thing as chaos. In an orderly universe, everything follows specific laws that result in patterns that can be seen in nature—cause-and-effect being the most obvious. In humans, patterns are powerful. They're also addictive. How many unconscious patterns do you follow every day that you're not even aware of? Do you take the same route to work so often that you miss the last ten minutes of the drive, and then suddenly find yourself pulling into the parking lot wondering how you got there?

Many people tell and re-tell their story so often that they're not even conscious of doing it. They're completely oblivious to the people they're alienating by unloading all their sorrows on them. They're also not aware of how strong a pattern or habit it's become for them. The most dangerous part of an addiction is when the affected person doesn't *know* they have an addiction. That's when they usually do the most harm to themselves. Such is the case with those people who are addicted to their story. They have no idea the amount of negative energy, words, and beliefs they're sending out into the universe that can only return to them more misery.

How could anyone be addicted to feeling miserable, sad, alone, and helpless? Easy. It's familiar. When we feel a certain way for a long time, it becomes our default energy set-point. It becomes our "normal." In the unconscious person, the human psyche will cling to this set-point of miserable (but familiar) territory, rather than risk a temporary imbalance to reach a new set-point. It also perceives this change as a "death" of the self, and as we're all naturally wired for self-preservation, it won't go willingly. So, their lives end up being a recurring pattern that looks something like: That "person" did "it" / or "that" happened to me at "that" time, which means I can't be/do/have (fill in the blank).

PASSING THE BUCK

There's another benefit for clinging to your story. You get to blame others. It protects people from the pain of having to take responsibility for their choices. Yes, a relationship may have been abusive, but if you look back you can probably find a few friends or family members who said, *"Don't marry that guy!"*

Making yourself a victim keeps you stuck in the small (i), your ego. It loves to makes excuses for perceived "failures." It's always somebody else's fault. Somebody or something else is in your way and you're powerless to change that. So, it's an easy out to sit there and do nothing. The high price for victimhood is giving up all your power to a person and/or event that never had any power over you in the first place. You get the benefit of sitting on a pedestal and claiming you never made a contributing mistake in any of these circumstances, and as a result, you end up with a life of inertia. Blaming others is like going through life with one foot on the gas and one on the brake. Moving beyond your small (i) into your true (I) means taking full responsibility for your thoughts, choices, and resulting life experience. In return, you get to use that power to change everything and anything, because you've not given any of it away. Full responsibility and full power will always be a package deal.

MOVING FORWARD

That's not to say that you shouldn't have compassion for yourself. Remember, we're all doing the best we can with the knowledge we have at the moment, even those awful people who did all those "things" to you. There is definitely a time to grieve and release an experience emotionally. It's essential to healing, but so is moving forward. Getting beyond a painful experience takes trust. It means taking the next step, even if you can't make sense of the experience right now. It's like being on the monkey bars as a child, clinging to one rung with both hands. You had to let go at some point to swing to the next bar and move forward.

Even so, it's in that moment of open space, feeling suspended in time, that you're not sure if your hand will catch the next rung. That is where we all need to trust the guidance of the universe and know that it will be there for us—that the next stepping stone will appear just as our foot breaks the surface tension of the water. That's what life is: a moment-to-moment, endless stream of death-defying acts, although we were never in danger for a second. It only felt that way.

A NEW PICTURE

The best way to let go of your story is to simply release it. Realize that you create a brand-new story every single minute of your life in the NOW. That's all there is. Your life isn't so much a novel with a single beginning, middle, and end as it is a long-running TV show, and every single episode is its own, brand-new story airing moment to moment. The best part is you get to constantly recast, rewrite, and perform every single one of them. If you didn't like the last episode, you'll get another chance to change the scene, then another, and another. You can't feel stuck if you've got a lifetime of opportunities to write many stories!

Reframing your story also helps you release it. That means sitting down and taking stock of all the negative experiences that have been keeping you stuck. Author Napoleon Hill said, "Every adversity, every failure, every heartache carries with it the seed of an equal or greater benefit." Remember, this is a universe based on balance. Nothing perceived as "bad" can come to you without an equal or greater amount of "good" in it. Perhaps if your crazy boss had not fired you, you never would have moved to another city and found a job making more money . . . and a new relationship!

This perspective helps to remove the sense of victimhood, but also allows us to see how we participated in creating our negative experiences. Perhaps you weren't "guaranteed" a raise at work, but went ahead and bought a new car anyway. It's not the company's fault that you're "underpaid" now. The flipside of this exercise can be painful, but it's also powerful. It's the part that gives you your power back when you see how you've had a hand in writing your story.

Perpetrators or Partners?

It's a challenge to reframe the negative experiences in our lives to find the good, but it's always there. Always. It's tougher still to take responsibility for our choices. Perhaps the biggest challenge is in dealing with the people involved in these experiences: the "perpetrators" who did all those terrible things to us. If you're brave enough to do this exercise and put your life under a microscope, you'll find that you've never really been a victim. That's great news. If there's never been a victim, then there never was a "crime," and without a crime, there can be no perpetrator. If there are no perpetrators in your story, then who are these people, and what purpose do they serve for you?

Remember, it's your story and you're writing it. Your life is a mirror image of you, reflecting back every energetic signal you've put out into the universe. That includes every circumstance and every person. Like energy attracts like energy. That means that, on some level, you were an energetic match for all your so-called perpetrators. You drew them and the resulting circumstances to you. If part of your story deals with someone else's selfishness, then it's important to ask yourself where you have been selfish in your life. If someone cheated you, where have you been cheating others or perhaps, yourself?

Every situation and person we encounter is an opportunity to learn more about ourselves. We're so quick to criticize others for their faults, but according to the old catchphrase and the universal Law of Attraction, "You spot it, you got it." Knowing this, we can see that every person who comes into our lives in a positive or negative way is truly our teacher. They're mirroring back to us a part of ourselves that we're not usually conscious of. Not only are we receiving a lesson, but we're also giving one to them. In every relationship, we're both teacher AND student. That's a gift! These people that we used to see as selfish or hurtful are signaling us to look inward to examine why we're attracting these types of people—so we won't keep making the same mistake. Our enemies are our friends. Once we understand the game of life on these terms, we can have compassion for ourselves and others.

To help heal these types of old wounds, I've used a visualization I call "Soul Lessons." I imagine I'm sitting around a large table with all the people who have hurt me most deeply in my life. We're there to write the script of my life. As I go around the table, I hear each one of my "soul mates" explain to me their role in my life and the valuable lesson they've chosen to teach me. They've volunteered to teach me these lessons in the clearest and sometimes most painful way so that I can move beyond my limiting beliefs and have a wonderful life. That's what they want for me. With genuine love and devotion, I hear them share their stories. If you do this for yourself in a nonjudgmental way, you'll be surprised at what comes through for you. Perhaps a "life partner" decided to be your cruel college professor who ridiculed your artwork so you'd have the courage to believe in yourself, regardless of opinions. Maybe another chose to be your cheating business partner so you'd understand how to keep a better eye on your finances. If you stay open, this simple exercise can fill you with gratitude and provide profound release.

REALITY CHECK... GOODBYE TO YOU

✓ The sequence of life events we've experienced up to the present moment we call our "story."

✓ We become stuck when we identify with our story and assume past events will predict future circumstances.

✓ Your story is simply the outcome of choices you have made, based on your beliefs at different moments.

✓ Because you can change your beliefs, you can change your story.

✓ People can become addicted to the sympathy or attention they get from telling their story repeatedly, and unconsciously draw more negative energy to them, creating self-fulfilling prophecies.

✓ Many people prefer to cling to their story, rather than experience the temporary upheaval of positive change, because feeling miserable has become familiar to them.

✓ Clinging to our story allows us to make excuses so we don't have to move forward.

✓ When we call ourselves victims, we give others the blame . . . as well as all of our power to change our circumstances.

✓ In order to have complete power over your life, you must claim total responsibility.

✓ In a timeless, now-centered universe, it's impossible for a previous event or person to hurt us. It's our misperception of it that we keep replaying in our minds that carries the pain.

✓ We can reframe any incident to find the greater good in it and change our perception.

✓ Our lives are not novels with a set beginning, middle, and end. We re-write a new episode moment to moment as a complete story unto itself.

✓ Because the universe is a mirror to our lives, the people who hurt us are our teachers. Their presence in our lives tells us to fix something amiss in our belief system.

✓ Let go of your story! Those who go through life looking backward will eventually run into a wall!

FOOD FOR THOUGHT

Reframing the Story

Take time below to write down some experiences from your "story" that you've been hanging onto. Write down your original perception of how things happened. On the following line, write down how you may have contributed to creating the negative situation. On the last line, list the good that came out of it. By reframing your story, you release the identity of being a victim and the limitations that go with it. Do this for as many situations in your life as you feel are holding you back.

Example:

1. *I haven't been able to get ahead because of the financial mess from my divorce.*

2. *I agreed that we should charge our last three vacations and I let him handle all the finances.*

3. *Even though it's a mess, I'm learning to manage my own money and become independent.*

Living in Advance

A great way to re-write your story is to actually write it! In the space below, write how you'd like your day to go tomorrow. Begin with waking up, and go through your day, listing all the things you'd like to happen with the people and situations you plan to encounter. So much of our creation in life comes from our expectations. If we expect to have a lousy day, the universe isn't going to stand in our way. It's going to get to work. Expectations are very powerful. When you write them down, they affect your subconscious in a different way. Look through your ideal day, as you've written it and see how and where you actually have the power to makes the things you want to happen, actually happen. Maybe that means being nice to your ex-wife *first!* Each night, try to intend the next day, visualizing it exactly as you'd like it to go and see what happens.

_____

_____

_____

_____

_____

_____

_____

_____

_____

CHAPTER 7

A LIFE IN PICTURES
THE POWER OF VISUALIZATION

"What is now proved was once, only imagined."
—**William Blake,** British poet and painter

"Live out of your imagination instead of out of your memory."
—**Les Brown,** author

"I saw the angel in the marble and carved until I set him free."
—**Michelangelo,** sculptor

In an energy-driven, attraction-based universe, what you see is what you get. Whatever your attention is focused on is what's developing in the unseen and working its way into your personal reality. For most of us, what we're seeing are the movies and images we create in our minds about the things we want and, more often, don't want.

A THOUSAND WORDS
We've discussed the power of our thoughts quite a bit, particularly when it comes to the words we speak. By the time the words leave our mouths, however, we've already had the thought that created them. In almost every case, that thought came in the form of a picture or an imagined visualization.

If I speak the words "Grand Canyon," what happens for you? You don't see the actual words in your mind. You instantly visualize the image those words represent. If you're afraid you'll be overweight for the rest of your life, you don't see that string of words parading across your mind. You see an image of yourself, sitting on a park bench, hobbled over with gray hair and a cane, feeding pigeons and looking like you're about to die from loneliness . . . and *then* you say, *"I'm afraid I'm going to be like this for the rest of my life."* Because our mind's imaginings carry the emotional charges that lead us to speak, it makes one mental picture worth more than a thousand words.

FROM ACTOR TO AUDIENCE

Because we think primarily in pictures, our mental movies can run away with us, often displaying the worst-case scenarios in vivid detail. When used consciously, visualization can be an extremely powerful tool in creating positive change in your life. In fact, visualization has been an essential tool in creating the accomplishments of the world's greatest artists, athletes, and even scientists. The problem for most of us is that these mental movies can seem so real that we get completely lost in the action. We become an audience member, a passive observer of them. We forget that we're the writer, director, and star of this movie, and that it is *only a movie.* When our perspective changes from being the artist to the audience, we begin to believe what we're seeing, and if it happens to be a horror film, there can't possibly be a happy ending.

It's your job to maintain creative control of your mental movie studio. Nobody else thinks in your mind. That means you can create the most vivid, sensory-rich, exciting visualization of the outcome of any situation, far beyond what you would normally think possible. These kinds of visualizations are even more powerful than affirmations because you participate in them. You can step inside of them and, from an imagined environment, create a real *experience.* (There's that word again.) Through the power of BEING in your visualization, you can come to KNOW something through experience and imprint upon the cells of your body what it ought to be. What you create in your virtual world, you bring into your material world. There's a reason visualization has become the habit of champions. This phenomenon was first tested and proven with athletes.

REAL WORLD RESULTS

NASA had been using a training device in their Apollo program called Visual Motor Rehearsal (VMR) for years. It wasn't until the U.S. Olympic team hired psychologist Denis Waitley, Ph.D. in the 1980s to incorporate it into their athletes' training programs that it became shockingly evident how powerful visualization was. Part of the training included connecting track and field athletes to specialized biofeedback equipment. They were told to run their events, but only in their minds. They were instructed to visualize, as clearly as possible, how they would look and what they would feel during the actual competition. The results showed that the neural transmitters and muscles the athletes would normally use to *physically* run the race all fired at the same level of exertion and in the same sequence, even though they never left their chairs. As Dr. Waitley said, "If you've gone there in the mind, you'll go there in the body."[24]

This is why professional athletes in all sports still use VMR as part of their training today. Athletes and even dancers take their bodies through endless courses of repetitive motion to engrain these physical demands into their muscle memory. Yes, the cells of your body do indeed have their own memory. After enough repetition, they can call upon the extreme amounts of strength, speed, and endurance they need in an instant without even having to think about it. This is also due in large part to their VMR sessions which have constantly strengthened and deepened the neural pathways in their brains that control these actions. *That's because the brain cannot tell the difference between a vividly imagined and a real life event.* The effect on our minds and bodies is exactly the same in either case.

DOERS & WATCHERS

To further illustrate this point, a study was done at Harvard Medical School in 1994 where volunteers were taught to play a five-fingered note pattern on a piano. They played this pattern for two hours each day for five consecutive days, while a second group just imagined playing the pattern and hearing the notes. At the end of five days, the neural pathways, or brain maps, for the groups were examined. As expected, the brain maps required for these actions showed significant strengthening in the group that actually played the notes. The pathways for the group that only imagined playing the instrument had also grown . . . to the same extent.[25]

Whenever we imagine doing any activity, not only do we become more dexterous, but we also become stronger as a result. A 2004 study done at the Department of Biomedical Engineering at the Lerner Research Institute in Cleveland showed that volunteers who were given a specific finger exercise program experienced a 53% increase in strength during the duration of the test. Amazingly, a second group that only imagined doing the exercises experienced a 35% increase in muscle strength![26] As if that isn't incredible enough, a similar study done in 2007 showed that volunteers who just watched the group that was physically exercising experienced a 32% increase in strength.[27]

Research has also shown that our strength gains come in direct proportion to the amount of effort we imagine exerting. The stronger the weights we imagine lifting or the greater amount of effort, the greater our strength gains will be.[28] An equally impressive study at the University Hospital Schleswig-Holstein in Germany showed that stroke patients who watched men and women perform routine functions, such as drinking a cup of coffee or peeling an apple, made significant improvements in conjunction with their regular rehabilitation when compared to the patients who did not watch these actions. MRI brain scans showed their neural pathways for these very functions were beginning to regenerate.[29]

The most powerful thing you can ever give anyone or anything is your attention. Always be mindful of where your attention is directed, whether it be a real or imagined scenario. Your ability to visualize can be one of your most powerful tools for personal change. Whether that change is positive or negative is up to you. Your mental pictures are energetic wishes. So be careful what you wish for. You *will* get it.

THE OTHER DIRECTION

As we learn to visualize what we want in our lives, we create and strengthen the neural pathways associated with those things. This system also works in the opposite direction. The neural pathways associated with whatever we *stop* visualizing or imaging literally weaken, become shallower, and fade away. It's like starving a bad habit to death. A good example of this is in people who studied a musical instrument, such as piano. Someone who was once quite good but hasn't played in 25 years will have lost a significant amount of their muscle memory required to play well. That's because the neural pathways associated with this activity will have begun to fade away. There's a scientific basis to "use it or lose it." You can use the power of visualization to speed your progress in two directions at the same time. As you visualize what you do want, you're creating new neural pathways, and sending out energetic signals to the universe that will cause it move toward you with great speed. At the same time, as you draw your attention away from what you don't want, those neural pathways shrivel, and their associated energy dissolves.

One of the most important skills they teach in racecar driving school is how to get out of a skid. With NASCAR speeds reaching just under 200 miles per hour, that's an essential skill to have. Even at domestic speeds, we've all been behind the wheel on a rainy or icy road and felt the terror of being out of control. This is the same feeling we can get when we're caught in a barrage of negative thoughts and images. We feel like we're spinning uncontrollably, quite literally caught in the skids of life.

Anyone behind the wheel of a car that's out of control *always* does the wrong thing. We look straight at the tree, brick wall, or ditch that we're headed for. That's okay. That's a reflex, but 99% of the time, it sends us straight into a crash. Even though you may be skidding off to the left, the key is to look to the right, instead. *Always look in the direction you want to go*, no matter where your car is headed or how fast it's taking you there. It feels counter-intuitive, but once a driver focuses on where he wants to put his car, his hands on the steering wheel will follow wherever his attention is directed and he'll get back on course.

When we're in the skids of life, we always seem to focus on what we fear. As we say mentally, *"Keep it way! Keep it away!"* we just move faster and faster toward it because we're giving it our attention and energy. *The key is to always look at where you want to go* no matter where you are in life. It can seem a bit jarring to do a complete mental 180-degree turn, but that's what you have to do. Use the exercises from the chapter on consciousness to snap yourself out of the skid and ground yourself physically in the now and then create a new vision. Look at where you want to go. Then, you'll be racing toward the finish line and not the tree!

Reality Check... A Life in Pictures

✓ Our thoughts come to us predominantly as mental pictures, not so much as specific words.

✓ You are not a passive observer of your mental movies. You are the writer, director, and star of them. You can choose the movie you're playing anytime.

✓ Consciously created visualizations with lots of vivid, sensory-rich detail are very powerful creative tools.

✓ Visualizations allow you to BE in the state or situation you desire and create a KNOWING for yourself without having to manage all the "real world" details.

✓ Visualizing how you want your body to be helps its cells record this state of BEING in their memory and set about manifesting it.

✓ Your brain treats a vividly imagined event exactly as it would a real world event. It cannot tell the difference, as it responds only from your feeling in the moment.

✓ The most powerful thing you can ever give anyone or anything is your attention. Be aware of what you're focusing on, in life and in your mind!

✓ What you image and give your attention to strengthens associated neural pathways in your brain. Withdrawing attention from something causes the associated pathways to fade away.

✓ When you're in a mental skid, always look at where you want to go. Ground yourself, then look in the opposite direction. Give your attention to what you want!

FOOD FOR THOUGHT

Setting the Stage

Some people are great at visualizing. Others find it more challenging. The key is to put yourself in the center of the action. Remember, you're not watching the movie. You're starring in it. It's the difference between what inspirational author Eric Butterworth calls just imaging and IAMaging. When you simply imagine, you're a spectator. With IAMaging, you're saying to yourself, "*I AM here. I AM this or that.*" Big difference. Don't see yourself in that size-8 evening gown. BE in it and feel how the fabric flows across your body. Does it have a texture? Hear the voice of your best friend approaching you at the party telling you how incredible you look. The more real you can make a scenario, the more feeling you'll summon, and the more energy you will create. In the spaces below, set the stage for your visualization. Write out all the sensory detail as completely as you can. Then close your eyes, and let this scene wash over you. Take at least ten minutes to allow the good feelings to fill you up to overflowing. Soon, you'll be able to visualize quickly and easily.

My visualized scene is: _____

_____

Visual Details:

Me _____

Other people _____

Environment _____

Sounds:

_____

_____

Tactile Senses (physical feeling):

_____

_____

Smell / Taste:

_____

_____

Out in Left Field

A great way to remove negative mental pictures is through collapsing them into another image. When a negative picture comes up, see and hear it crumpling like a sheet of paper into a ball and toss it into a trash can, or hear the grind of putting it through a paper shredder. Throw a rock at it and hear it shatter like glass as the pieces fall out of your field of vision. Hear the crack of a baseball bat as you hit it out into left field. See it racing out into the distance, getting smaller and farther away from you as it bursts into a tiny puff of smoke. These kinds of exercises quickly diminish the power of negative images and help you redirect your attention. You'll be surprised how powerful they are.

CHAPTER 8

MYTH & MADNESS

THE MYTH OF BEAUTY / THE MADNESS OF WEIGHT LOSS SURGERY

*"You don't love a woman because she is beautiful.
She is beautiful because you love her."*

—Anonymous

*"You can take no credit for beauty at sixteen, but
if you are beautiful at sixty; it is your soul's own doing."*

—Marie Stopes, author

*"Beauty isn't worth thinking about. What's important is your mind.
You don't want a fifty-dollar haircut on a fifty-cent head."*

—Garrison Keillor, American humorist

Living in the western world, specifically the United States, has historically provided opportunities that someone might not have in most other countries. The blessing of this has always been a person's opportunity to find his own path in life and become anything he chooses. The rags-to-riches success stories of some of the world's wealthiest industrialists and entrepreneurs are a testament to that. The downside of living in a country anchored in capitalism is that it often leads to unbridled consumerism. In order to keep the economy from stagnating, people need to keep spending money. How do they keep spending money if they can afford all their basic needs? Easy. Convince them to buy things they *don't* need.

KEEPING UP & CASHING OUT

The bedrock of the entire advertising industry is founded on this very principle. The research methods they use to coax money out of our pockets today lies somewhere between surreptitious and subliminal. In the 1950s, advertising was straightforward. Products were sold for their functionality and convenience. They swept the floor, baked a meatloaf, or mowed the lawn easier and faster. Products were sold on the premise that they could make your daily routine better.

By the time the 1970s arrived, something had changed. The two-income household had materialized and, suddenly, people had more money to spend. In order to get that money moving into the market, the advertising industry took a new approach. The dawn of concept advertising had come. Realizing you can't sell someone something they know they don't need, the drive became to *create a need* for the product. If someone doesn't actually need the product, then what do you have to sell? You don't sell the product. You sell the "idea" of the product or the assumption of what the product will do for a buyer. Enter the era of advertising psychology. Instead of products being sold on the basis of speed and convenience, they were now being promoted as chic, sophisticated, sexy, and professional. Human personality traits were being attached to material products, and the assumption was that you could take on those characteristics if you bought "the right" pair of sneakers, dress, car, or perfume. It's no wonder some people have 30 pairs of shoes. They're still searching for "the right" pair. This change in perspective was beyond significant for society. No longer were we being told a product could make our daily routine better, but that the product could make **us** better.

So strong was the pull of this new advertising angle that many manufacturers didn't even have to show the actual product in an ad anymore. If an average-looking guy walked out of a club with a beautiful woman on his arm in a TV commercial, that was reason enough to buy a particular brand of toothpaste, breath mints, or cologne. Ultimately, Americans find themselves in a race to "keep up with the Joneses," always "needing" the bigger house, faster car, more powerful computer, latest cell phone gadget, and so on. We're afraid of being perceived as not as good or less successful because we don't have all the newest "stuff." It's a cycle of constant comparison, a trap of "not enough-ness" that forces us to keep up with the neighbors while cashing out our bank accounts.

BUYING BEAUTY

Nowhere is this phenomenon more successful than in the health and beauty industry. Considering the fact that Americans spend on average $60 billion on weight loss programs[30], $19.5 billion on gym memberships[31], $10.5 billion on cosmetic surgery[32] and $7 billion on cosmetics[33], it's easy to see there's lots and lots money to be made in making you feel inadequate.

A study done by *SELF Magazine*, in partnership with the University of North Carolina at Chapel Hill, showed that 65% of American women between 25 and 45 have some type of distorted relationship with food, from banishing carbs to skipping meals. Nearly 67% of the women in this age group are trying to lose weight at any given time. This total did not even include the 10% of women in the U.S. who have been diagnosed with clinical eating disorders such as anorexia and bulimia. When you put it together, three out of four women behave abnormally around food. Some would rather be unhealthy than overweight, as 13% opted to smoke solely because it suppressed their appetites.[34]

What is going on?

EPIC PROPORTIONS

As the saying goes, when someone tells a lie long enough, they'll begin to believe it. The truth is the earlier and more frequently we're exposed to lies, the easier it is to believe them. By the time concept advertising hit and both parents in a household were working, the TV became American's new babysitter. For overwhelmed parents with tight schedules, it became all too easy to sit the children in front of the TV and let them be. As we've already discovered, a picture is worth a thousand words in the mind, and a child's subconscious is fertile ground for advertising images. Many of those images came from seemingly harmless products like toys.

Over the last six decades, Mattel's Barbie doll has been the benchmark for classic American beauty: Caucasian, blond hair, blue eyes, and a coveted hourglass figure. Barbie's iconic status among generations of girls has led grown women to seek cosmetic surgery to look more like their favorite toy. When it comes to Barbie's body, however, you're likely to need much more than plastic surgery—maybe a magic wand—to get a figure like that. On the

50th anniversary of the Barbie doll, *BBC News Magazine* decided to adapt Barbie's proportions to a real woman to see what her figure would look like. A woman standing 5'6", maintaining her 28-inch waist, would have to be 7'6" to get Barbie's proportions. At that height, her hips would measure 40-inches and her bust 37-inches. If the real woman kept her height of 5'6", she'd end up with a waist of just 20-inches, a bust at 27-inches, and hips at 29-inches. Researchers at the University Hospital in Helsinki Finland said that if Barbie were a real person, she'd lack the 17-22% body fat required to menstruate.[35]

Odd Man Out

It might seem funny to picture a real life, 7'6" Barbie. Even as absurd and unattainable as they know it is, women still strive to reach this ideal, or something like it. Supermodels Cindy Crawford, Tyra Banks, and media mogul Oprah Winfrey have all gone on TV without so much as a stitch of makeup, hair extensions, or body binders to show that the idealized, perfect woman doesn't really exist. Even with the magic trick of commercial beauty exposed, women still choose to believe the illusion. They may not be playing with Barbie anymore, but that doesn't mean they're still not incredibly influenced by the media. Studies show that a woman only needs to be exposed to as little at 30 minutes of TV programming before it alters her perception of her body.[36]

I believe a large part of this hypnotic attraction to perfection lies in a desperate need to belong. One of the most visceral human needs is a sense of belonging or inclusion in a group that supports and understands us. It gives us a sense that we are important to something bigger than ourselves and that we are not alone in the universe. Human beings are social creatures and belonging is intrinsic to our very nature. When we feel like we don't belong, we experience isolation and loneliness that can be crushing and even physically painful. It's the very reason certain religious sects use the practice of shunning members as a form of punishment. Jail wardens know that the only thing worse than being in prison, is being in solitary confinement in prison. Isolation *hurts*. We know the media spins their Hollywood mirage through fog lenses, perfect lighting, airbrushing, and photo manipulation. Still, the images are very powerful and, when in Rome, we want to do as the Romans do. It's the same reason everyone goes out and buys the same red coat that happens to be in fashion one season. The coat may cost a week's salary. They may not even like the color red, but if enough people begin wearing it, they'll have to have it, too. That's not fashion. It's the need to belong.

The style of celebrities, models, and sports stars is even stronger because we respect them, idolize them, and feel like we know them. They're not all wearing red coats, but they have a universal style and appearance that we strive to emulate. When you never see anyone who looks like you in magazines or on TV, you feel insignificant, left out, and unimportant. So many times, we feel our only choices are to remain invisible or try to join the in-crowd by becoming like them. It's the polite form of self-hatred. Comedian Whoopi Goldberg used to create a poignant version of her younger self in her stand-up routines where she would pull a sweatshirt over her head and pretend it was her long, beautiful blond hair. The documentary, *Good Hair*, produced by comedian Chris Rock, followed African-American women and girls as they endured caustic chemical treatments and expensive straightening procedures to achieve hair with more Caucasian features. At its extremes, finding our place in the world can cost us dearly physically or financially, but that's because, to us, the cost of not belonging is even higher.

THE UGLY TRUTH

It's not enough to look like the media images we see. We want all the things that looking like that is supposed to bring us. Everybody knows the "beautiful" people have easier lives and get all the opportunities. At least, that's what it seems. It's always the beautiful (aka, skinny) girl who gets the guy and the high-powered job in the movies. It's always the macho man who saves the day. The ugly truth about most of the so-called beautiful people is that they're all struggling with their own set of issues. Someone's outer appearance has nothing to do with their self-image. Most models don't even think they're pretty. Many actors and actresses are terribly insecure. We're all struggling with the same issues in one form or another. The supposed good life of being a beautiful person isn't what we think is. It isn't even for those who are living it. These are just a few comments 'traditionally' attractive women often make.

- *No empathy*: I'm not allowed to have real problems. People think because I'm skinny or pretty, I'm just being a drama queen.

- *Shallow relationships*: Finding true friendships with depth is hard. People think because I'm pretty or skinny I'm superficial, and those are the kinds of people I attract.

- *No female bonding*: Other women see me as competition, so I can't establish deep friendships with them.

- *No Intimacy*: Men never approach me. They're intimidated by me. The ones I do meet only date me for my looks.

- *Aging Obsession*: My beauty is my power that gets me what I want in life. As my beauty fades, so will the opportunities.

The prettiest girl in the room can also be the loneliest girl in the room. Yet when we're down, it's easier to think someone else is living the problem-free, jet set life. It's often been said that if everybody's troubles were put into a bag and mixed up for a drawing, you'd take your own back in a minute.

The Invisible Man

When it comes to body image and weight loss, one segment of the population remains completely invisible: men. For decades, women's bodies have been objectified, and as a result, they've faced the worst kinds of social rejection if they didn't fit the desired mold. Because of this, weight and body image was seen as a "woman's" problem, and as such, most interventions were aimed and marketed toward them. It was assumed that men could be "fat and happy." They didn't care about belonging, looking good, sexual attractiveness, or self-image. They just weren't self-conscious enough to care about such things. The problem was that they did care, but to talk to someone about it would have meant risking being seen as unmanly.

It was previously thought that only 10% of anorexia and bulimia patients were men, until Harvard University released a study in 2007. It was the first national study of eating disorders that used a population sample of 3,000 adults. The researchers were shocked to find 25% of those with anorexia and bulimia, and 40% of the binge eaters, were men.[37] It's also been understood that boys who go through school participating in sports where weight is a crucial competing element, such as wrestling, swimming, gymnastics, and horse jockeying, are more prone to having food and weight-related issues as adults.

Measuring Up

It's clear that men suffer from the same body dysmorphic perception as women do when it comes to the media. If you're not over six feet tall with a 48-inch chest, carry the confidence of an action hero, and look like a movie star, then you're seen as less of a man. Adding insult to injury is the new wave of "metrosexual" masculinity. If a guy is lucky enough to actually be tall, dark, and handsome, it still doesn't fit the bill. He's got to be manicured, pedicured, perfectly coiffed with the right hair care products, and in the most strategically-coordinated clothes. In major metropolitan areas, the pressure on men to be as aesthetically beautiful as women has become daunting. Like women, these ideals are coming from a media onslaught aimed at men. Images of the "perfect man" that no one can live up to clearly damage a man's self-image. What wasn't known until recently, however, is that sexualized photos of the "ideal woman" affect men in an equally negative way.

A study done at the University of Missouri found that male college students had more feelings of body self-consciousness and anxiety *after* they viewed sexualized cover photos of women from magazines such as *Maxim* and *FHM*. Contrary to popular belief that men often find these kinds of photos titillating, the study showed it left them with a feeling of inadequacy that they couldn't measure up to being with such a woman.[38]

BIGGER IS BETTER

In response to feeling inadequate, many men try to measure up by overcompensating for what they see as a masculinity deficiency. Instead of dieting, many become obsessed with exercising and bodybuilding. Because it looks to outsiders like they're "just a health nut," many men can hide their eating disorders and body image issues behind a lifestyle that appears acceptable on the surface. In the book *The Adonis Complex*, author Harrison Pope, M.D. gives accounts of men who quit high-level jobs and lost relationships because they interfered with their excessive workout schedules. Some men would nearly panic if they had to miss a workout, and instead, would lift the furniture in their hotel room or office.[39]

It doesn't matter what you're talking about: in America, bigger is always better. It's no wonder that when men don't feel like they're enough, they resort to building themselves up to beyond-grotesque proportions. Like anorexia in reverse, men who suffer from body dysmorphia constantly see themselves as much smaller than they really are, and become driven to achieve muscle gains that are physiologically impossible without risking their health by using steroids. It's a phenomenon that's informally been dubbed "bigorexia" in gyms around the country.

A study published in the *Harvard Gazette* asked male students to choose from a set of photos the kind of body they wanted to have. Consistently, the men chose photos of physiques with 30 lbs. more muscle than they had on their own frames. Ironically, when females were asked to choose the most attractive men from the photos, they regularly chose the models with 15-30 lbs. *less* than what the men thought was ideal.[40] Even with women telling men it's not necessary to be that big, they too can't seem to pull themselves out of the media-driven illusion that they're not good enough. Who could blame them? They had their own version of Barbie.

AVERAGE JOE?

The G.I. Joe doll for boys rolled off the assembly line in 1964. At the time, he had an average physique. If he were a real man standing 5'10", he would have had a 32-inch waist, a 44-inch chest, and thin, 12-inch arms. By 1991, his waist had shrunk to 29-inches and his arms had grown to 16-inches. By the middle of the decade, the G.I. Joe Extreme action figure, standing 5'10", would have had a 55-inch chest and the largest biceps of any bodybuilder in history.[41] Even action figures for nostalgic superheroes like Batman and Superman are sporting nearly deformed muscular proportions today, carrying all sorts of negative body images for young boys. These are the icons they respect, the benchmark they're measuring themselves against. This is what a "real man" is for them.

THE THREE C'S

When we're constantly exposed to images of seemingly perfect people, our next logical assumption is that their lives are perfect, too. When God was passing out the brains, beauty, and billions of dollars, they got in all the right lines. It's easy to look at a thin, sexy woman or handsome, successful man and assume their lives have been without struggles. How else could they have accomplished such amazing things? On the contrary, considering what we've learned about the number of dysfunctional households in America, I'd say the odds are very, *very* good that they've accomplished wonderful things *in spite of* their upbringing. Knowing this teaches us never to assume that someone else's life is a cakewalk. It also gives us proof that we too can overcome our own obstacles and achieve our dreams. In fact, it's the people that *have* overcome great odds in life that we find the most inspiring. Think about it. Would you rather watch a movie about a man who inherited his family fortune and traveled the world, or read the story of a single mother of five who went to night school to become a lawyer and was eventually elected to Congress? It was actress Mary Tyler Moor who said, "If you've never had anything bad happen to you, then you can't be that interesting."

So much of our own suffering in life is self-inflicted, usually when we make assumptions about the lives of others. We experience it when we engage in what motivational speaker Paul Pearson called the Three C's. We constantly **compare** ourselves to others in regard to body image, salary, or accomplishments. We **compete** with others on these levels to establish a sense of superiority and self-worth. If we feel we're on the losing end of that competition, then we **complain**. In her book, *Tripping the Prom Queen: The Truth about Women and Rivalry*, author Susan Shapiro Barash shares interview data that reveals 80% of women admitted to competing with other women through their physical appearance.[42]

Because your body and life are just the computer printout of what's happening in your own mind, life is really a "one sum" game. It begins with you, ends with you, and is truly ALL about you. Another person's apparent beauty, success, or failure has no impact on *your* life. None. By engaging in the Three C's, you generate more feelings of shame, anger, and inadequacy, telling the universe to create more situations where you can feel shameful, angry, and inadequate. When interviewed, most winning athletes usually say their only real competition was with themselves. They never paid any attention to the swimmer in the next lane or driver in the other racecar. Their only goal was to create a new personal best performance by focusing on what they needed to do in that moment. That's how the race of life is structured . . . and won. Your only competition is you, and you become a champion based on your own terms.

CUT TO THE QUICK

When we're constantly comparing ourselves to others, we always think we're losing out on the great job, the house, the car, the guy or the girl that someone else is getting that's rightfully ours. We want change, and we want it fast. Who doesn't? Life is too short. It's this sense of insecurity and urgency, however, that can cause us to not trust the natural order and flow of life. Our biological clocks are ticking. There's no time left, so we make the mistake of overriding our intuition with intellect, leading us to find a quick fix that isn't always in the best interest of our desires or our health.

Gastric bypass surgery, or the Roux-en-Y procedure, has been around since the 1960s, but it's only been in the last 15 years that it's become a hot topic in the media. During that time, the cost of a gastric bypass became more affordable as an increasing number of Americans began to be classified as obese. You couldn't turn on your TV without seeing the latest news anchor, pop singer, or other celebrity touting the benefit of this "life-changing" procedure. Talk shows were parading guests across their stages who'd lost hundreds of pounds in an alarmingly short period of time. The before and after images of these people were astounding. Who could argue that a real solution to weight loss and been found? No one. At least, not initially.

BAD TO WORSE

By 2006, the number of surgery patients would eventually grow to about 140,000 per year.[43] During that time, post-operative patients began exhibiting uncharacteristic addictive and compulsive behaviors for substances and actions they'd previously had no interest in. Some began shopping themselves into bankruptcy. Others began smoking, gambling, or having a large number of sex partners, while others gravitated toward drinking.

In a phenomenon known as addiction transfer, it became clear that if the emotional root of a patient's weight gain was not properly addressed before surgery, they would be driven to find another substance with which to numb their pain. It was a classic situation of treating the symptom and not the problem. In an effort to find a quick fix, no one seemed to recognize that the weight was the *effect* of the problem and not the problem itself. The medical establishment wasn't quick to acknowledge this issue. Some surgeons insisted that having gastric bypass surgery didn't "make someone an alcoholic," completely missing the point. While the subject needs further study, a presentation at the American Society for Bariatric Surgery Association's annual meeting in 2006 stated 30% of patients experience an addiction transfer after surgery.[44] Even as late at 2011, online post-op gastric bypass blogs are full of heartbreaking stories of people drinking two bottles of wine in a sitting, affairs and broken marriages, thousands of dollars in shopping debt, and even illicit drug use.

JUST A DROP

The attraction to alcohol seems to be the most prevalent addiction transfer for gastric bypass patients, and there is a physiological reason behind it. Dr. John Morton of Stanford University has performed many gastric bypass surgeries himself. When he began hearing accounts from patients who were having serious reactions to small amounts of alcohol, he became suspicious. He even heard anecdotes from patients who'd drank only one glass of wine and received a DUI.

Morton conducted his research through the Stanford University School of Medicine and the results were sobering. After drinking just five ounces of red wine, gastric bypass patients experienced a blood alcohol content level (BAC) of 0.08% as compared to the non-surgery participants' level of 0.05%. The gastric bypass patients took 108 minutes to return to a BAC of zero, while the control subjects reached the sober state in 72 minutes.[45]

In a follow-up study in 2010, published in the *Journal of the American College of Surgeons*, Morton focused on the BAC levels of patients prior to and after surgery. Using the same amount of wine, Morton discovered that in just three months after surgery, a patient's BAC was already above the average level, measuring 0.059%. By six months post-op, the BAC of patients was rising to 0.088% with the same amount of wine and in the same amount of time. That's more than triple their BAC prior to surgery, which measured only 0.024%. At the six-month mark after surgery, it was taking patients nearly 1½ hours to reach a sober state that only took them 49 minutes prior to the procedure.[46]

These results showed definitively that gastric bypass patients have a significantly altered ability to metabolize alcohol. It also explained why alcohol was such a danger in transfer addiction. Patients became inebriated faster and it took longer to return to a sober state. It was as if their bodies were hot wired for alcohol and even a single drop could open the door to a much more serious situation than dealing with excess weight.

DANGEROUS TRADEOFF

In gastric bypass surgery, the stomach is reduced to about the size of a small egg by creating a pouch at the top. This pouch is then connected to the middle portion of the intestine (jejunum), bypassing the rest of the stomach and the upper portion of the small intestine (duodenum). The smaller stomach greatly reduces the amount of food a patient can consume. Hence the assumption that fewer calories eaten translates into more pounds lost. That may be so, but the balance of biological metabolic processes is more than simple math. It also means that since alcohol no longer has to pass through the full length of the digestive tract, it enters the bloodstream much faster. Since food absorption takes place in the small intestine, which has now been largely circumvented by the surgery, it becomes more difficult for the body to take in the proper amount of nutrients. This is also due to the drastically reduced amount of food patients can consume after surgery, usually just one ounce. This is crucial because every substance the body uses to keep itself alive comes through the digestive system. If it's being bypassed, that does mean fewer calories are being consumed, but also far fewer nutrients are being absorbed. Post-operative patients must follow strict supplementation guidelines for life when it comes to all their vitamins and minerals including vitamins A, D, E, B12, and especially protein.

BARIATRICS & BUSINESS

With the beauty myth operating at full force through the media, bariatric surgery made the leap from medicine to marketing when the National Institutes of Health (NIH) decided to lower the body mass index (BMI) standards in the late 1990s. BMI has traditionally been used to assess a healthy weight in comparison to height. In 1998, the NIH lowered the maximum healthy BMI weight limit from 27.8 to 25. It was said the change was made to correspond with weight ratios from the World Health Organization (WHO) and to reflect increases in mortality of people with a BMI over 25.

Overnight, 29 million people had a weight problem . . . at least on paper. Added to the total number of Americans that were already dealing with a legitimate weight issue, 55% of the population at the time, or 97 million people in the nation were now considered overweight.[47] Under the new guidelines today, a *normal* BMI is between 18.5 and 24.9. Anyone beyond 25 is considered overweight, while those over 29.9 are classified as obese. By today's standards, a person standing 5'3" and weighing 141 lbs. is overweight as is a man at 5'11" weighing 215 lbs. Classifications like these were hotly debated in public health circles at the time, as were they in professional sports. Knowing that lean muscle mass weighs considerably more than fat, virtually every professional athlete from basketball, football, and even gymnastics was now considered overweight. As laughable as it sounds, I don't think anyone would call NBA player Shaquille O'Neal obese. They might just find themselves slam-dunked head-first through the basketball hoop.

Suddenly, it was easier for hundreds of thousands of people to qualify for weight loss medications as well as surgery. At virtually the same time, the number of bariatric surgeries began to rise dramatically. According to the American Society for Bariatric and Metabolic Surgery, the number of bypasses being done has risen six-fold since 2001. In 2009, 220,000 procedures were performed.[48] The demand for the surgery has become so great that hospitals across the country are creating specific centers for bariatric surgery within their facilities. In the last several years, independent "quality assurance" organizations, and even insurance companies, have been bestowing dubious Awards of Distinction on the centers to enhance their credibility and promote the surgery as a weight loss intervention.

Most recently, a major pharmaceutical corporation has petitioned the Food and Drug Administration (FDA) to lower the required BMI for patients seeking gastric band surgery. The Lap-Band, as it's known, is considered less invasive because it uses a plastic band to partition the stomach off instead of cutting and reshaping it. To currently qualify for gastric band surgery, a patient must have a BMI of at least 40, or 35 with one coexisting condition such as diabetes. Today, about 15 million Americans meet those criteria. Allergan, the company proposing the change, has requested that the eligible BMI be dropped to 35, and go as low as 30 with one additional health problem such as high blood pressure. Under the revised limits, a man standing 6ft. tall and weighing just 225 lbs. would qualify for the surgery—strange, considering current BMI standards would only put him 37 lbs. over his weight limit. After taking effect, an additional 27 million Americans would qualify for the surgery—a total of 42 million potential patients.[49]

The cause for alarm from the weight loss support community has been that the modified requirement standards for surgery will encourage even moderately overweight Americans to naturally gravitate toward solutions that seem quicker with easier access--especially ones their insurance will pay for. It's another incentive to avoid the battle to get insurance companies to pay for extended psychological and emotional interventions. In an interview with *The New York Times*, Dr. Louis J. Aronne, obesity expert at Weill Cornell Medical College, said, "It would be kind of ironic if people have access to surgery and not medical therapies, where they can go from Weight Watchers to surgery and have nothing in between."[50]

Projection analysts expect these changes to create an explosion in gastric band surgery revenue, reaching $390 million by 2016.[51] All this in spite of a recent study at the European School of Laparoscopic Surgery in Brussels that revealed 40% of gastric band patients experienced major complications, with 50% having to have the band removed and 60% requiring more surgery.[52] The pharmaceutical company insists the physicians were not trained to install the device properly. In either case, it's important to know that the same corporation also manufacturers Botox, breast implants, and dermal fillers.

STARTING EARLY

While TV advertising for Barbie dolls and actions figures have been aimed at children for decades, so has promotion for some of the most nutritionally-void, artificial food substances ever manufactured. Children's TV programming is littered with advertisements for candy, soda, frozen treats, sugared breakfast cereal, and virtually any product that contains high fructose corn syrup. Add to that the unhealthy state of public school lunches and it's no surprise that our children now mirror the obesity problem in our adult population.

This situation has created the perfect opportunity for the pharmaceutical corporations to begin promoting bariatric surgery for adolescents. The subject has always been controversial, but increasing numbers of children have been undergoing surgery since 2001. The exact number isn't known and national statistics are extremely difficult to find. Even so, the *Archives of Pediatric & Adolescent Medicine* report that 771 adolescents under the age of 20 received bariatric surgery in 2003.[53] When you consider that a recent study by the University of California, Los Angeles (UCLA) showed that 590 adolescents between the ages of 13 and 20 received bariatric surgery between 2005 and 2007 in the State of California alone[54], it becomes clear that the popularity of surgery as a weight loss intervention among children is quickly rising.

WHAT LIES AHEAD

Heated debate continues over whether a 14-year-old child can comprehend the consequences and responsibilities that come with bariatric surgery, and how the outcome will radically change the way he or she will live the rest of their life. That's if things go *well*. No one has even begun to investigate the threat of addiction transfer in adolescents once the companionship of food is no longer available as a coping mechanism. Common sense tells us that teens are at an extreme risk because drugs and alcohol are immediately available on many high school and college campuses.

The most recent concerns surrounding adolescent bariatric surgery were presented at the American Association of Pediatrics' 2010 annual meeting. Data presented by Dr. Diana Farmer, Chief of Pediatric Surgery at Benioff Children's Hospital at the University of California, San Francisco, showed that teenage girls who had gastric bypass surgery carry a high risk of having babies later in life with neurological defects such as spina bifida. This was due to the girls' inability to absorb vitamin B6 and folic acid, two essential nutrients for neurological formation in the fetus.[55]

Bariatric surgery for adults is controversial enough, not to mention the ethical questions that arise when adolescents enter the equation. How does it make sense to impose such a radical physiological change on a body that's only half way through its growing phase and a psyche that hasn't even begun to mature? Any pediatrician will tell you that when it comes to treating children, they're not "little adults." Medical care is administered to them in a very specific way because they are not living inside their permanent adult body, yet. That's why we have doctors who treat only children. Does it make sense, then, to put a child through an adult surgical procedure and expect them to just adapt without radically different outcomes? It's important to note that, as of this writing, bariatric surgery for adolescents between 13 and 17 has not been FDA approved but the pharmaceutical corporation that manufactures the gastric band is lobbying for the change.

Yet, the rush is on for more children to have bariatric surgery even though we have no idea what the long term ramifications will be. Some doctors are reporting receiving up to ten phone calls a week from parents seeking the surgery for their children, some as young as 8-years-old.[56] These well-intentioned parents are being driven by media hysteria that constantly declares the "adolescent obesity epidemic." Riding the same wave, pharmaceutical corporations swoop in as the savior that will rescue their children from diabetes, high blood pressure, stroke, cancer, and an early death. What parent wouldn't want to protect their child from such danger? The truth is the numbers just aren't there to prove it yet, and who's willing to take the risk with their child to do so?

SAME APPROACH

Critics will often point to studies such as the one recently published by the American Heart Association. It was the longest study of adolescents with gastric bypass surgery performed by the Cincinnati Children's Hospital Medical Center. The study followed post-op patients under age 19 for two years to examine if heart structure and blood pressure improvements were still stable. They were. What the study also shows is that while the children did lose weight, the average BMI after two years was nearly 40—still classified as obese.[57] That means a 5'4," 14-year-old girl who participated in the study would still weigh 235 lbs. two years after surgery. What was really accomplished?

A study published in the *Journal of the American Medical Association* showed that a group of adolescents that underwent gastric banding surgery lost up to 50% of their excess weight, while those who participated in a "lifestyle change" program did not.[58] It's no wonder. The lifestyle change program consisted of counting calories, exercise, keeping a food diary, and limiting the amount of TV viewing. If this approach hasn't worked for millions of adults, why would it work for adolescents? There was no spiritual or emotional component to the program, yet we've known for years that the core of a weight problem is an emotional one. How could these children be expected to succeed where adults with more discipline and self-knowledge have not?

HIDDEN SIGNALS

We need to be very careful of the message we're sending to our children. A teen who is presented with the option of bariatric surgery by a parent isn't necessarily hearing a concerned plea for their health as much as a signal that they're not okay just the way they are right now. Yes, there are long-term health ramifications that come with being obese, but the keyword here is "long-term." I've yet to hear of a 17-year-old who dropped dead of obesity. There is cause for concern with our children, but no cause for alarm. Not yet. To subject an adolescent to surgery that changes their life so drastically, when they cannot possibly grasp the lifelong consequences or has not received the proper psychological and spiritual interventions, is irresponsible and unethical. I'm not suggesting that all bariatric surgery is bad, but I am joining the ranks of an increasing number of physicians who are raising their voices to say it should only be used as an absolute last resort where the life of a patient is in imminent, not "projected," danger.

Even seemingly benign cosmetic changes in our children's appearance are beginning to reveal a darker side. While not conclusive yet, initial studies are beginning to show that orthodontia, particularly in young people, is having lasting negative effects. Nickel alloys in stainless steel braces have been known to create heavy metal poisoning, resulting in depression, severe weight loss, and behavioral problems. Removing wisdom teeth for strictly aesthetic reasons is being linked to pituitary and thalamus gland malfunction, and uncharacteristic cravings and eating patterns. As an osteopathic physician, I have studied the meridians that are the energetic superhighways of the body, connecting every organ and tissue to each other. When these energy pathways are disrupted by removing any part of the body or forcing it from its original alignment, imbalance of some kind always occurs. This is why I believe dentistry and orthodontia should never be cosmetic but medically necessary, and always carefully considered beforehand with a holistic dentist for all children, as well as adults.

A Grain of Salt

When it comes to needing an authority on anything, the media is the last place to go. What's good for us today will threaten our very health tomorrow. It wasn't that long ago when eggs became the new forbidden food. You couldn't turn on the news without hearing how the cholesterol was going to send you to an early grave. Avoid them like the plague. Several years later, eggs were terrific for you again . . . well, just the whites. The yolks had too much fat. Now, the whole egg has fallen back into favor. What changed? It wasn't the egg. The media has done this 360-degree switcheroo with red meat, whole milk, and virtually every other food and personal care item you can possibly think of. The fear machine that is the media, that's constantly creating insecurity and pushing perfectionism, is the last place anyone should go for an authoritative view on anything—especially real health or beauty.

In another classic about-face, the media ran to broadcast a recent Japanese study that flies in the face of their fear-driven, excess-weight-means-early-onset-disease horror stories. The study showed that those who were slightly overweight by the age of 40 actually lived six to seven years *longer* than people who were thinner.[59] The moral of the story is, if it's in the media, always take it with a grain of salt. Trust yourself, especially when it comes to choices than will change your life or the life of someone you love forever.

If you're looking for the secret to real beauty, remember how the universe works. When you learn to see beauty in everything, then *you* will become beautiful . . . and beautiful things will come to you.

REALITY CHECK... MYTH & MADNESS

✓ Our economy is sustained by constant consumerism. In order to keep people buying products, marketing campaigns must create an internal sense of inadequacy in the consumer.

✓ Concept advertising tells you that a product won't make your life better. It will make *you* better.

✓ The media-driven images of beauty that we focus on, even casually, have a direct effect on our emotional state and self-image.

✓ Seemingly benign images such as toys, dolls, and action figures easily skew a child's image of what a "normal" body looks like.

✓ Women who are defined as traditionally beautiful experience many hidden obstacles in their lives as a direct result of their physical appearance. This includes difficulty in establishing deep, meaningful relationships.

✓ Men make up an unexpectedly large percentage of those struggling with weight, yet they are easily forgotten in weight loss interventions aimed almost exclusively at women.

✓ Over-sexualized images of women make *both* men and women feel inadequate about their bodies.

✓ A false sense of beauty easily leads you into the Three C's: compete, compare, and complain.

✓ An increasing number of bariatric patients are experiencing addiction transfers and other complications.

✓ The long-term effects of bariatric surgery on adolescents are unknown at this time.

✓ *Always* consider all the lifelong consequences of weight loss surgery, and be sure it's only used as a last resort.

✓ When you learn to see the beauty in everything, then you will become beautiful.

Food for Thought
Art School

One of the best ways to change your perspective on beauty and body image is to adopt someone else's. Take some time and do an internet search on classic paintings and sculpture. It's fascinating to look through the eyes of an artist, at a time when media influence did not exist, and experience their perception of what was considered truly beautiful. How might our standards of beauty change if all we had to look at was each other in our most natural form?

Below is a list of paintings of women and sculptures of men that are universally considered exquisite human forms by art historians for their composition and symmetry. I don't see any size-2s or Mr. Universes in this crowd.

PAINTINGS
Flaming June: Lord Frederic Leighton

Birth of Venus: Botticelli

A Bathing Place: Albert Moore

Female Nude Reclining on a Divan: Eugene Delacroix

The Fortune: Guido Reni

Female Nude and Pianist, Jean Honore Fragonar

Cleopatra: Gian Pietro Rizzi

Venus Anadyomene: Titan

The Birth of Venus: William Adolphe Bouguereau

The Source: Ingres Jean-Auguste-Dominique

Actaea-The Nymph on the Shore: Lord Frederic Leighton

Union of Earth and Water, Peter Paul Rubens

SCULPTURE
Apollo Crowning Himself: Antonio Canova

The Dying Gaul: Unknown

Apollo Sauroktonos: Praxiteles

Perseus with the Head of Medusa: Benvenuto Cellini

The Youth of Antikythera: Euphranor of Cornith

CHAPTER 9

HOW DO I LOOK IN THESE GENES?

THE REVOLUTION OF EPIGENETICS

*"Our own physical body possesses a wisdom
which we who inhabit the body lack.
We give it orders which make no sense."*

—**Henry Miller**, *author*

*"Our bodies are our gardens.
Our wills are our gardeners."*

—**William Shakespeare**, *playwright*

"Our bodies are apt to be our autobiographies."

—**Frank Gelett Burgess**, *artist*

After years of becoming frustrated with diets, everyone has a moment where they stare into a photograph from the past and think something like this: *"My whole family has struggled with weight. I guess it's just genetic. I'm a big-boned person. It's hereditary. I've never been thin in my life. It's not in the genetic cards for me."* Since our elementary school science classes, we've been taught that genes determine every facet of our human life, from hair and eye color to weight and personality traits. It's as if we come into the world with a pre-recorded blueprint of a specific biological story that will eventually unfold, and there's nothing we can do about it. If you happen to struggle with obesity or even develop cancer, that's just too bad. You drew the short straw from the genetic pile. You'll have to tough it out and hope for better luck in the next life.

TRUMP CARD?

Luck? Knowing what we know now about physics, energy, the power of thought, the Law of Attraction, and the dynamics of an *orderly* universe, it's obvious that luck does not exist. Nothing is random. Every effect has a cause. Could a particular gene assist in the creation of obesity or caner? Yes, but what *creates the gene* that created the condition in the first place?

Humans are so hard-wired to believe that genes are the be-all-end-all of their existence that we've become the victims of our own biology. Remember, when we assume the role of a victim, we give away all our power to change anything. We take on the attitude that this is "just the hand life dealt me." In addition to being resigned, we've also terrified ourselves with genetic theory. If our mother and sister had breast cancer, or our father and uncle had heart attacks by age 45, then we become convinced that will be our fate, too. In years past, the discovery of so-called "breast cancer genes" have driven many women to surgically remove their perfectly healthy breasts as a *precaution* against the "inevitable." Nothing trumps the genes.

A NEW DEAL

That simply isn't so. On average, only seven in 100 women carry the so-called breast cancer gene. Even so, not all of them will develop cancer[60]. So, what makes the difference?

We know we create our entire lives and everything in them. That includes our bodies *and* the genes that give rise to them. Everything means EVERYTHING. Everything is energy, directed into form by our thoughts and feelings. If that was not so, then the concept of free will would not exist, and I assure you that it does. In addition to quantum physics, a revolutionary new field of research known as epigenetics[61], pioneered by cell biologist Bruce Lipton, Ph.D., is confirming scientifically what we've always known about our lives intuitively and spiritually. It's proving that if we don't like the hand we're dealt, we can shuffle the genetic cards and create a new deal. In fact, we're doing it all the time. We just never knew it.

Our DNA and genes exist in the nucleus of the cell. Conventional wisdom has told us that the nucleus is the "brain" of the cell. It controls all functions of life. We've learned earlier that the universe is created from the inside out—from microcosm to macrocosm. That being understood, the cell also has a respiratory, digestive, circulatory, and other functional systems just like its larger counterpart, the body. Our organs carry out these functions for us. In the cells, organelles do the same job. Common sense tells us that if we remove the brain from a living organism, these processes will immediately stop, and it will die. Research has now proven that if the nucleus is removed from a cell, it continues to live and carry on its normal functions ... *with no DNA or genes in it!* This discovery has shown us that the nucleus cannot be the brain center of the cell and that genes do not control the cell or its expression. If the nucleus and its genes aren't controlling the cell, what is and where is it?

THE SKIN YOU'RE IN

In high school biology, we learn an embryo has three layers: an ectoderm, mesoderm, and endoderm. Every single organ, tissue, and fluid of our bodies is developed out of these three layers. Interestingly, the outermost layer, the ectoderm, gives rise to just two: the skin and the brain/nervous system. Your skin and brain are inextricably linked. Your skin is the interface between you and your environment. If you're cold, it senses that and shivers to generate more heat. If you're embarrassed, it senses that and causes you to blush by rushing blood to its surface. If you're nervous, you perspire or get goose bumps. Your skin reads the environment and tells your cells what to do. In similar fashion, it is the membrane or skin of the cell that reads signals from its outer environment and tells the inner parts what to do. The brain of the cell is its skin or membrane.

ABOVE & BELOW

The building blocks of the body are proteins. It's what gives us our structure, but if we were just protein, we'd be like statues unable to move and stuck in place. A protein needs a specific signal to alter its electrical charge and cause it to change shape, open, or close, just like your garage door opener needs a specific signal to open or close. It's this

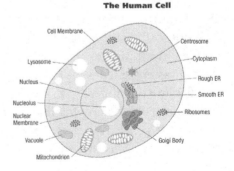

The Human Cell

constant shape-shifting that animates our cells and bodies.

The membrane of a cell is not smooth. It's covered with thousands of tiny **receptors** that look like antennae. Their function is the same as our five senses. There's one to match every conceivable stimulus from its environment. Complementing each receptor is an **effector** site that looks like a manhole cover on the street. When a receptor receives a signal that matches it, that signal is sent below the membrane, telling the inner cell what's going on and how it needs to respond. Because the receptor is a protein that has just received a matching signal, it changes the shape of its lower half that extends beneath the cell membrane. Like pieces of a puzzle, the new shape of the receptor fits perfectly into the lower half of the effector, which opens up its cover on the cell membrane to allow the requested proteins to escape and carry out the appropriate response. No nucleus necessary. No genes.

What's in Store

The nucleus is just the warehouse of the cell. It contains all the spare parts to keep it going in case one of the organelles wears out. That's why a cell with no nucleus will eventually die after a few months; not because the nucleus is the driving force of life, but because there will be nowhere to go for resources once the old parts need replaced. The nucleus also comes into play if the receptor relays a signal to the inner cell and the specific protein to carry out that request isn't available.

The signal will travel to the nucleus, the store of spare parts. Inside, it finds the chromosomes, which are protecting 25,000 genes, each in their own protein coating. Just like the surface regulator, the signal travels up the entire strand of DNA until it finds the protective protein that matches its signal. Like a key in a lock, the protein changes shape, opens, and allows the gene it's protecting to be copied. The new gene is released into the cell, received by the effector and sent out into the body to complete the request.

All of a Sudden

The truth is we're all walking around with genes that have the capacity of creating virtually every disease and condition known to man. Unless those genes are **specifically requested by the matching signal**, however, it's *impossible* for them to come into play. Genes for cancer, Parkinson's disease, obesity, and any other condition are completely powerless unless they're activated by the matching signal. Without the signal, these genes remain locked in their protective protein coatings which keep them inactive.

If just having a specific gene caused cancer and you possessed it, then you should have expressed that condition from birth, just like your blue eyes or brown skin. Clearly, this is not the case for the vast majority of people. Someone might live problem free and then develop cancer at 35. Does it make sense then to blame the gene? The cell is using its sensory receptors to read its environment and respond to the signals we're sending it through our own sensory receptors . . . our five senses. **Our entire human biological system (body) is run by the physical awareness or sensation of its physical environment**. What is awareness and sensation of an environment? Our *perception* of that environment!

That's why it's essential for me as a physician to go back into the past with my patients and investigate when there was a significant change in their environment. Was there verbal abuse, sexual abuse, a divorce, abandonment, a horrible accident, or some other event that caused a change in perception of their world or circumstances? What thoughts and feelings are they harboring from these incidents that are causing a negative signal to be repeated in the cells of their bodies? Emotional states that cause illness have often been carried for years, long **after** the incident itself has passed and **before** sickness arrives. This is why I always say that, in medicine, there is no such thing *as "all of a sudden I felt this pain,"* and, *"then one day I noticed a lump,"* or, *"out of nowhere came this fatigue."* Every effect has its cause, and nothing happens out of the blue.

POINTS OF PERCEPTION

The behavior of the cell is NOT programmed. It's changing its response moment to moment because of the signals we're sending it, based on the perception of our environment through our senses. Perception and environment, however, are two *different* things. Our genes are constantly adjusting to fit our perception of the environment we "think" we live in. In fact, the raw material of our so-called "fixed" genes comes and goes every six weeks.[62]

What is a perception? It's just a belief. Your genes don't know that a particular incident happened 30 years ago. If you're still hanging onto the negative emotions and beliefs from it, your genes are responding as if it's happening now.

To Each His Own

If you and I go to a movie, it could be the best film I've ever seen and you could think it was awful. The difference isn't in the movie. It's in our perception of it. This is why an external event like a divorce is *never* a "first cause" for anything. Millions of people get divorced, but not everyone puts on weight after the fact. If that were the case, everyone who ever had a similar experience would have the exact same response. Common sense tells us that's not true. If the experience is the same, the only differing factor is *the person having the experience* and how they're *perceiving* it. It's the difference between, *"It will be tough for a while, but I'm glad we're divorced. Now this opens the door to someone who treats me with respect,"* and, *"I feel so humiliated by that cheater. How could I be so stupid to have missed it? I can't trust anyone anymore."* It's these false perceptions and the emotional signals they generate that dictate the genetic functions of our cells. How we relate to any issue **IS** the issue.

This is why your girlfriend can eat three slices of pizza and still fit into her favorite jeans. If you're sitting across from her, nibbling on your tiny sliver, thinking about all that saturated fat that will come back to haunt your waistline, you're sending a very specific signal to your genes to *"hold onto the fat"*! The points of perception between you and your friend are very different, and you're telling your body two different things . . . and getting two very different results.

I know of a family with four sisters, three of whom died of cancer before they were 50. The fourth sister, who never developed cancer, is now approaching a healthy 70. Was it luck of the draw that kept her alive or her perception of how her life would be different?

Circle of Life

Knowing what we know about our thoughts moving energy to create matter, and ultimately how that process is reflected in our bodies, we can say the "real" Circle of Life goes like this: An EVENT occurs that we OBSERVE or experience, which is filtered through our PERCEPTION of it, after which we form a JUDGMENT as to whether it is "good" or "bad," which leads

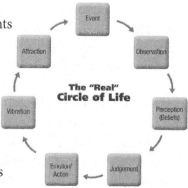

to an EMOTIONAL REACTION, that results in a specific VIBRATION being sent out into the universe, that creates an ATTRACTION for another matching EVENT, and so on.

It seems like a lot of steps, but this process happens in a fraction of a second in every facet of our lives. This is why it's essential to **not** trust your physical senses if you want real change in your life. If you constantly see yourself as overweight and unhealthy, you're sending that directive to your cells. As you believe, so shall you be . . . literally.

This is the true creative process of life and it's impossible to turn it off. We're always re-creating and in constant communication with our bodies. The nature of life is to be creative and grow, so we can't stop this process. We can't necessarily control an event, but *we can control our reaction to it*. We can intervene in the creative process by becoming aware of our perceptions and *choosing an action* instead of jumping into a reaction. When we consciously decide how we want to see an event, we deliberately choose how we feel, and the rest of the creative process comes under our control. This is why all the sacred sages of the past have stressed non-judgment. See things and have wonderful experiences, but don't label them, especially negative situations. To do so incites a strong reaction, which creates energy that may bring back to you something you do not want, even on the cellular level.

When it comes to your body, think of yourself as the captain of a ship. Down below, in the bottom decks, is your loyal steerage crew, your cells. The crew keeps the fires of the engine stoked and executes every demand the captain sends them. Even though they cannot see where they're going from that far below deck, they trust the captain implicitly and carry out his commands based on the directions he's sending them. They have to trust him; otherwise they would drive the ship right onto the rocks. That's why it's important to understand the world of illusions that affects your senses so you can consciously choose the signal you want to send to your crew based on the direction you want your body and your life to go!

MOTHER KNOWS BEST

So our genes are not performing based on what's happening in our environment, but on what we *think* is happening in our environment. As we've seen, the perceptions or beliefs we carry through life come largely from our parents. We also know that we get 50% of our genes from our mother and 50% from our father. In fact your parents, particularly your mother, were selecting your genes while you were still in the womb, through the same process based on their perceptions of their own environment. If an expectant mother lives in a dangerous, violent or abusive environment, she will be choosing the appropriate genes for her unborn child that will allow it to "survive" in the environment it is about to be born into.

A great example of this phenomenon is the story of the Dutch hunger winter of 1944. In that year, the Nazis had invaded Holland and chose to divert all the food resources from the region back to Germany. Thousands starved for months and many died. If a woman was pregnant during this period, she was sending a very specific request to her own genes and those of her unborn child: *Food is scarce. Hold onto every single nutrient you can find to survive.* For the next six decades, the children of the Dutch hunger winter and their descendants showed significantly higher rates of blood pressure, obesity and metabolic syndrome.[63]

Our genetic connection to our mothers can't be overstated. How much more unified can you become with another human being than to have their blood running through your prenatal veins? It's also been discovered that the mitochondria of the cell has its own set of DNA. The mitochondria are the engine of the cell, and provide it with the energy it needs to carry out its functions. Unlike the nucleus, 100% of the DNA contained within the mitochondria comes from the mother.[64] Think about that. All of the DNA contained in the engine or driving force of the cell comes from your mother. This is why when patients begin to investigate for subconscious roots to disease or obesity, I quite often suggest they start by looking at their relationships with their mothers.

CONSTANT CHANGE

It doesn't matter whether we've adopted subconscious beliefs from our parents or created them on our own, we *can* change them. It always helps to understand where our beliefs come from, but it's not always necessary to have that information to change them. Even if you don't know specifically why you carry extra weight, you can begin to feel healthy and thinner now by creating that kind of *environment* for yourself and acting AS IF your desire is already accomplished. Wearing sexy clothes that complement your figure, being in the company of uplifting, healthy people, and splurging on a dessert every now and then is sending a very specific signal to your cells . . . so is wearing caftans and filling your grocery cart with "diet" versions of your favorite foods. You don't always need all the answers to start moving forward now. In fact, it's essential that you not wait for them. Do the investigative work, but begin sending a new signal to your cells ASAP!

Once you choose new signals, you begin selecting new genes. A famous study was done years ago in which researchers extracted a gene involved in learning and intelligence from a mouse. As a result, the mouse became less intelligent and did not learn as quickly. The story the media ran was that there was now undeniable proof that there were genetic limits to how smart a person could be. What they didn't publicize was the last half of the study. When the mouse was put into an *environment* that was highly stimulating, he completely overcame that deficit.[65]

This is proof enough that predisposition to a certain condition is a far cry from predetermination. The mind is not in the body. The body *is in the mind* and the mind is in something much, much larger. You have the power over the unfolding of your own life. There are no victims. Yes, you can look gorgeous in your genes . . . if you *choose* the right pair.

REALITY CHECK... HOW DO I LOOK IN THESE GENES?

✓ Our genes are not fixed. We select them based on the thought-driven / emotional signals we send to our cells.

✓ We send signals based on the perception of our current environment.

✓ Perceptions about our environment are our *beliefs* about it.

✓ If we perceive we are in a stressful, angry or dangerous environment, we will select genes that correspond with these negative emotions and eventually express themselves in our physiology.

✓ We can turn genes on and off by consciously selecting the messages we'd like to send to our cells—positive, loving thoughts.

✓ When be become conscious of how we perceive our environment, we can change it.

✓ Many of our perceptions come from our parents, even before we were born. Investigating our parents' perceptions can be valuable tools in changing our own.

✓ You don't always need to know the "why" of your perceptions. You don't need all the answers to begin sending your cells new signals now.

✓ The best way to send new signals is to feel good NOW. Feel what you want NOW. Act as if you had your desire NOW. Your cells are *always* listening.

✓ It doesn't matter if an incident happened decades ago. If you're hanging onto the feelings and emotions of it, your genes are responding as if it's happening now.

✓ You have control over the unfolding of your life and the expression of your physical body by your perceptions of yourself and the world around you.

✓ Predisposition to weight gain or any other physical condition is a far cry from predetermination!

FOOD FOR THOUGHT

Family Tree

Take some time to speak with family members, particularly your parents. If it's possible, ask questions about the environment your mother was living in during her pregnancy. See what her perceptions were of that environment and how they may have changed now. Speak with older siblings. Many times they can share memories of your early experiences that you're completely unaware of. Aunts, uncles and other extended family members can provide valuable information into why and how you see the world the way you do. These early life experiences may reveal unconscious beliefs or perceptions you hold about your environment. When you become aware of them, you can change them.

CHAPTER 10

THE PLEASURE PRINCIPLE

THE SELFLESSNESS OF SELFISHNESS

*"Why not seize the pleasure at once? How often
is happiness destroyed by preparation, foolish preparations."*

—**Jane Austen**, author

*"Nothing would be more tiresome than eating and drinking
if God had not made them a pleasure as well as a necessity."*

—**Voltaire**, philosopher

*"The secret of success is learning how to use pain and pleasure
instead of having pain and pleasure use you. If you do that,
you're in control of your life. If you don't, life controls you."*

—**Tony Robbins**, motivational speaker

Any time we want to heal and see real change in our lives, we must approach the situation from a place that addresses the body, mind, *and* spirit. Because evolution always moves from inner to the outer—microcosm to the macrocosm, it is essential that real healing and change begin at the innermost depths of our being, our Spirit. Spirit is your true identity. It's what you really are. We've talked extensively about your mind, but you are not your mind. Your mind is a tool. You use your mind to create your life. You are the power that chooses how to use that tool.

The problem with most medical, weight loss, and psychological interventions today is that they insist on treating the outermost layer of your being, providing care at the end of the creative assembly line instead of at the front. As long as the conveyor belt is in motion, you'll never get a different product if you're always working at the end of it. It's like treating the symptom instead of the disease. The body, in whatever its current manifestation, is just the symptom. Medicine is great at prescribing pills for symptoms, but if healing is to be permanent, a shift needs to happen at the Spirit level. From there, it will radiate outward through the mind and ultimately be gloriously manifested in the body. Whether it's permanent weight loss or healing from a terminal illness, the seed of healing is always planted in the soil of the Spirit first. *Always.*

SOUL FOOD

We can understand the material aspect of our bodies. We can even grasp the idea of choosing our thoughts. When it comes to Spirit, however, the definition seems to become a bit gray. It doesn't matter what you call it, your Spirit, Soul, or higher Self. It's the innermost part of you that only desires two things: the deepest love and the highest self-expression. When it comes to healing our Spirit, we have to *feed* our Spirit. How do we do that? We do it with pleasure.

All the things you've ever wanted to do, whether it's travel, sing, paint, take dance lessons, work with children, design jewelry, write a book, or play a better golf game, you want because they will bring you pleasure. These are the desires of your Spirit. They are the yearnings that call out in your quiet moments. *"THIS is who I really am!" "I know I can do that!" "I've always wanted to do that."* These things and activities are more than just fun. They fill you up with a joy that brings with it a sense of accomplishment and completeness. Remember, we are electrical, emotional, and vibrational creatures. True pleasure resonates with us on these intimate levels. Author and philosopher Joseph Campbell knew this when he advised, "Follow your bliss and the universe will open doors where there were only walls."

The pleasure principle is so vital in healing that I call it *Spiritual Nutrition.* We've already seen what heightened emotional states can do for the body on a cellular level, for good or ill. When we make a conscious decision to seek out pleasure on a daily basis and feed our souls, we put rocket boosters on our healing process. The power of pleasure cannot be overstated.

LIFE OR DEATH SENTENCE

One of the greatest examples of the power of pleasure comes from Dr. Bernie Siegel's classic book, *Love, Medicine and Miracles*[66]. A man named Arthur was a patient of Dr. Siegel's who had been diagnosed with advanced stage-4 cancer and was given six months to live. He was told to go home and get his affairs in order, and do his best to enjoy the time he had left. Dr. Siegel didn't expect to hear from him again.

Five years later, Dr. Siegel ran into Arthur in the grocery store. He was stunned. He told Arthur he was supposed to be dead and asked him what happened. Arthur replied, "Dr. Siegel, you probably don't remember what you told me, but you said I only had six months left to live and that it was important for me to make it the best six months of my life. I took your advice. I quit my job, which I never really liked. I went on a cruise, which is something I'd always wanted to do, and I began taking piano lessons, which was something else I'd always wanted to do. After six months, I felt so good I decided I didn't have to die. I've not been sick in the past five years, and I've never felt better in my life."

Out of curiosity, Dr. Siegel decided to check on many more patients he'd sent home to die. To his astonishment, he found out that 20% of his "terminal" patients were still living years later . . . and completely healthy.

WHAT ABOUT ME?

Normally, it would seem easy to pursue our bliss and indulge in things that bring us pleasure. What could be so hard about that? A lot. Feelings of guilt, misguided fear about being perceived as selfish, or just being too busy keep most people from experiencing real pleasure and feeding their souls. A Soul that's not fed is a Soul that starves. When the Soul begins to die, so does the body.

There's debate on this topic, but many respected physicians who have treated thousands of patients have made mention of a specific personality type that is common among women with breast cancer. These women tend to be very self-sacrificing, never taking any time for themselves. They're always running the kids to sports practice, organizing the PTA fundraiser, working overtime so a friend can take the day off, or canceling their plans to help a neighbor move into a new house. Under a veil of being extremely nice, these women tend to harbor unconscious resentment that no one ever does anything for them. They never get their own time, and feel lost in the shuffle. It's the energetic vibration of suppressed anger that ultimately contributes to their diagnosis.

SELFLESS SELFISHNESS

Selfishness gets a bad rap in our society. Whenever anyone does anything for themselves strictly for pleasure, it's viewed as selfish . . . especially if you're a woman and you "should" be taking care of someone else instead of yourself. Here's some valuable advice: Your life is all about YOU as far as the universal Law of Attraction and your cells are concerned. Your cells are responding to how YOU think and feel. Participating in things that give you pleasure can *only* make you happier and healthier, and that will definitely make you a better mother, wife, daughter, sister, Girl Scout troop leader, or birthday party organizer.

When I stress the importance of pleasure to patients, I often hear the same response. "Yeah, but I'm the only one who can _____." As wonderful as it might be to think the world will stop if we're not constantly scheduling other people's lives, it won't. Nobody's indispensible and the world *will* go on turning. There's nothing noble about falling over after a double work shift or dropping dead at a church bake sale. When you are selfish enough to feed your own soul in the ways that are most important to you, it is the most selfless thing you could ever do for those you love.

FEEL GOOD FOOD

For those who struggle with weight, the last thing they allow themselves to take pleasure in is food. It doesn't matter what we eat. If we're eating unconsciously to fill a void or numb our pain, we don't really taste the brownies, pizza, or whatever else we're consuming. We miss all the pleasure of the experience— the aroma, texture, and flavor of our food. While never scientifically proven, it's been assumed for years that the people of France remain the thinnest in Europe because they allow themselves to take full pleasure in their eating experiences. They have their occasional bread or pastry, and wine at every meal. They revel in the richness of their cuisine and don't give calories a second thought. That's the key: their thoughts. Guilty eaters tell their bodies that they should be punished for eating something they enjoy and so the body responds by adding on the weight that it's expected to gain. When we fully engage in every moment of an incredible meal and we're feeling *good* about it, our bodies (and cells) process the food in a completely different way. You see, when we sit down to a piece of pie or slice of pizza, it's the taste, texture, and experience of our favorite foods that we really want. If we eat slowly, chew thoroughly, and allow delicious foods to reveal themselves to us, we become satiated much sooner. The first piece of pie tastes exactly the same as the third. When we really allow ourselves the pleasure of food, one piece of anything—and sometimes just a bite—is enough to provide the experience we were looking for. Call it quantum eating, but it's true. In fact, the French may be onto something, as they're ranked as the 128th most overweight country in the world. The United States is 9th.[67]

DEPRIVATION NATION

The other way we deny ourselves the pleasure of food is through deprivation. Anyone who's ever been on a diet knows that eating carrots and lettuce only lasts so long before deprivation explodes into overindulgence. The same thing happens when we consume all the fake diet foods that "taste like" chocolate, cream cheese, or cookie dough. Your body is smart and won't be fooled with engineered foods that, to be honest, just taste like the boxes they came in. Anyone who's trying to lose weight *always* has more success when they incorporate foods they really love into their diet and even splurge on the rich ones once in a while. We already know what happens in our body energetically-speaking when we're feeling good, regardless of whether that feeling comes from hearing a funny joke or enjoying a piece of birthday cake.

So often, when we're trying to do something good for our health, we restrict ourselves to food that we don't like. It's assumed that if something tastes bad, then it must be good for you! On the contrary, science has shown that humans have taste buds for a reason.

Two groups of test rats were put through an experiment on taste sensation. Both groups were fed a normal rat diet, but the second group received a tasteless version of the same meals. Within a very short time, the taste-deprived rats all died. During the autopsies, researchers could only find one cause of death: malnutrition.[68] It's clear that there is a physiological link between taste and health. If we do not enjoy the food we're eating, regardless if it's broccoli or brownies, we're absorbing fewer of its nutrients. Through your taste buds, your body is getting the signal that something "bad" is coming and gets prepared to reject it.

The same phenomenon appears in patients who are being fed intravenously or through a feeding tube. These patients often express a nagging hunger for taste even though they're presumably getting all their required nutrients. While more research needs to be done in this area, one thing is clear: In order to be fully nourished by our food, we must take pleasure in it.

RECIPE FOR SUCCESS

A lot of ingredients go into living a successful life and accomplishing the things we desire. There is no specific recipe, and you don't need one. The basic tenet is, if it brings you pleasure, then it's healthy and healing for you. If it doesn't, then it's not. There are some ingredients, however, that are fundamental to everyone. It's like building the perfect pizza. You can put whatever toppings and spices on yours that you like, but it's got to have the right crust and sauce for it to be a success.

National Geographic explorer Dan Buettner spent years traveling the world, and discovered that certain communities around the world enjoyed near-zero obesity and chronic disease rates, while their members lived an average of 100 years. Although culturally different, these communities, or Blue Zones[69], which were found in Greece, Japan, Italy, and even California, shared nine lifestyle characteristics that brought them great pleasure. These included having a **purpose** in life that gave them a sense of value. All claimed some sort of **belief system** in a grand design that was greater than themselves. They also had an extremely strong sense of **community** support through their **families** and **friends**. In Okinawa, residents belong to *moais*, or groups of five friends who are bound together for life. So important is this sense of community to our well-being that science has given it a formal name to study it: intersocial neurobiology.

LIGHTEN UP

Few things give us more pleasure than laughter. When was the last time you laughed yourself to tears? When we laugh, our whole body opens up and positive energy courses through every cell. When we want to change anything in our lives, especially our weight, we tend to take it far too seriously. Because we tell ourselves that we'll start enjoying life *when* we lose the weight, all the joy gets sucked out of our lives. We don't lose the weight. That "future" day never comes and we just end up having a big, miserable NOW. Being dedicated to changing your weight is always a great thing. Being serious about it is not. It's the difference between knowing two cookies **can't** undo four weeks of conscious, healthy eating, and feeling you might as well eat the whole bag because you've "blown it" again anyway.

Laughter really is the best medicine for anything we want to change in our lives. It's not just a metaphor. In 1964, famous U.S. political diplomat and author Norman Cousins was diagnosed with ankylosing spondylitis, a horrifically painful degenerative disease of the spine, and given a 1-in-500 chance of survival. Because the disease is considered incurable, this was basically a death sentence.

His homemade healing regime included watching old Marx Brothers films. He found that when we experienced deep laughter, he could get two hours of pain-free sleep each night. Soon, his blood sedimentation rate and white cell count (disease markers) were dropping significantly. Ultimately, he completely recovered from this "incurable" disease and shared his story in both the *New England Journal of Medicine* and his own book, *Anatomy of an Illness.*[70]

Laughter and the pure pleasure it brings are indeed powerful life changing elements. If they can help bring someone back from the brink of death, certainly they can be just as powerful in helping us lose weight. Amazing unseen magic happens inside our bodies when we experience pleasure. So give yourself permission to experience it. Let's learn to not take ourselves so seriously. Nobody else does!

REALITY CHECK... THE PLEASURE PRINCIPLE

✓ Your spirit, soul, or higher self is the part of you that seeks the deepest love and the highest self-expression.

✓ Our spirits seek healing through the pleasurable expression of their desires.

✓ Spiritual nutrition is even more important than diet when it comes to healing our bodies and lives.

✓ We feed our spirit with the pleasure of family, friends, humor, artistic expression, and intimacy, among other things.

✓ Selfishness is good when it means we consciously take the time to create pleasurable experiences for ourselves.

✓ Rejuvenating through pleasure enhances all of our relationships and is one of the most selfless things we can do for those we love.

✓ Your life is all about YOU. Your cells are always responding to the pleasure you are or aren't feeling in any moment.

✓ Eating consciously and allowing ourselves to deeply experience the aroma, texture, and flavor of the foods we love is a very pleasurable experience.

✓ When we eat consciously, we are satiated sooner and consume less, because it's the sensation of the food that satisfies us—not the quantity of it.

✓ When we feel good about what we're eating and taking pleasure in it, our bodies process the nutrients and calories in a completely different way.

✓ Our bodies absorb more nutrients from food when it tastes good!

✓ Strong social relationships are so vital to healing that science has given it a name for study: intersocial neurobiology.

✓ To take full pleasure in life, we must NOT take life so seriously . . . beginning with ourselves!

FOOD FOR THOUGHT

Pleasure Priorities

Most of us don't take the time to experience real pleasure, much less allow ourselves to think about it. If we actually stop to consider what really brings us pleasure, we might be hard pressed to come up with a list because it's been so long since we've actually experienced it. In the space below, list some small things that bring you pleasure—things you could incorporate into your life today, like gardening, a bubble bath, or getting a massage. Next to it, list bigger things you could plan for in the near future, like taking a cruise, riding rollercoasters, or a road trip with a friend.

Small Pleasures	*Big Pleasures*

Palate Pleasures

Choose a food item you *love*. No, it doesn't have to be traditionally healthy for this exercise. Just make sure that it's a single-serving portion. That means just one brownie or piece of pie, if that's what you're going for. Sit down in a quiet location with no distractions. Make sure your phone isn't going to ring, the TV is turned off, and you're free from disturbances. Use a watch or a timer to give yourself five minutes. Take the first full minute to really look at your food. Examine the color and visible texture. Look for things you may not have noticed before about it. Pick your food up and smell its aroma. Take in the scent like a connoisseur of fine wine. How many different scents can you pick out? Maybe it isn't just chocolate, but there's a hint of vanilla and hazelnut, too. If you close your eyes while doing this, your sense of smell will be enhanced. Then, take the first bite. Notice its physical texture. How does the aroma change once it hits your tongue? Is it richer, smoother? Does the flavor deepen? Chew each bite until it is a liquid before going onto the next. Make sure you take the **full five minutes** to finish this portion, and then check in with yourself afterward. How pleasurable was the experience? Are you satisfied? How was this conscious eating experience different from other meals for you?

CHAPTER 11

HEAD SPACE
THE MIRACLE OF MEDITATION

~~~

"Muddy water, let stand always becomes clear."
—**Lao Tzu**, *founder of Taoism*

"All of man's troubles come from his inability to sit alone,
quietly, in a room, for any length of time."
—**Blaise Pascal**, *French mathematician*

"You do not need to leave your room. Remain sitting at your table and listen. Do not even listen.
Simply wait. Do not even wait.
Be quiet, still and solitary. The world will freely offer itself to you to be unmasked. It has no
choice. It will roll in ecstasy at your feet."
—**Franz Kafka**, *Jewish novelist*

We know that everything is energy, directed into form by consciousness. Our consciousness can only take on the shape and nature of those things of which it is aware. If every physical thing, including human beings, is made of this same energy, then every material object must come from the same consciousness . . . and indeed, it does.

This takes us back to the principle of ONE. Everything is interconnected and comes from just one singular source. That source is the universal creative consciousness or God consciousness, as some call it. This great consciousness has just one goal: to know itself. It does this by manifesting into countless living creatures, people, places, and things that constantly give it new scenarios and experiences to be "aware" of, to learn and grow from. Consciousness is forever seeking expansion through an endless evolution of life experiences . . . including yours and mine.

ALL FOR ONE

There is no duality. There is no black or white, up or down, right or wrong, you or me. There are simply an infinite number of manifestations of the one creative process used by a singular great consciousness. How can that be when there are clearly 7 billion seemingly-different people on Earth? Think of it this way. When you receive an email from a friend, that message is not actually in your computer. It's not in any real singular location. It's floating out there somewhere in cyberspace. No one really knows where the internet as a whole exists. We just know that it's *out there* and there's only ONE. The internet is like universal God consciousness. It contains all the information we could ever want or need to live the fullest, most satisfying lives. Its information and possibilities of what it can do for us are endless. As human beings, we are like the individual computer terminals that reach out into this consciousness and download the information of our choice. What appears on the screens are the images and situations of our lives.

Have you ever thought of calling a friend and, just as you reached for the phone, that very person rang you up first? Have you ever had the feeling that a friend or loved one might be in trouble and need your help? Have you ever had a great idea for a clever invention, only to turn on the TV and see someone promoting the very same device? That's because we all share the same, singular consciousness—the very mind of God, within which all ideas, inspiration, and answers exist. Every person who has ever lived or will ever live exists not as an individual, but as an *individualization* of the one great universal consciousness, seeking to expand and grow through our separate experiences. This is why Christ declared, "I and the Father are ONE."

Consider the ocean. We may designate different areas of it as the Pacific, Atlantic, Indian, or Arctic, but the truth is that there's only one continuous body of water that covers the Earth. Across this vast ocean, trillions of waves rise and fall every minute. These waves are different from the ocean in the sense that we can see them peaking above the surface. Each wave may be larger or smaller in relation to others, but they are still connected to the ocean as a whole. In fact, each wave contains the exact water, mineral, and salt content of the ocean that gives rise to it. So as human beings, we *appear* different to each other but, in fact, we are all connected to the great ONE. We are created in its image and likeness, have access to all of its knowledge, and have never once been separated from it.

Mystery Solved

It's been said that universal consciousness, or God consciousness, is like a circle whose center is everywhere and circumference is nowhere. You exist within and are *an extension of* this endless consciousness. Because there is only ONE, it is whole. It is complete. That means it contains the answer to every question that could ever be asked. There are no mysteries. Every solution, whether it be to weight loss or world peace, exists right now within the universal consciousness that we are all using to create our lives. Nothing is ever hidden from us. That's why we are told to "seek and ye shall find." The answers we seek are available to us right now. The problem is that we don't seek at all, or keep looking in the wrong places.

Those places always tend to be *outside* ourselves. We want to jump right into our problems, roll up our sleeves, and begin "fixing" everything with an intellectual approach. More often than not, those approaches just leave us feeling frustrated when they eventually fail. The solutions to our problems are intuitive in nature, not intellectual. The power we possess through our connection to universal consciousness far exceeds our intellect, and we access it through the practice of meditation.

The Secret Place

For more than two thousand years, we have been taught to pray in the wrong direction. We have been taught to pray outwardly to a separate God, in a separate location, who may or may not, depending on his mood and whether we're living the "right" way, grant our wishes. This premise is simply not true, because it's built on duality—the idea that God is someone or something somewhere else, when we know all is ONE. That means the all-knowing universal God consciousness is not in a church, synagogue, or mosque. It's right where you are, **right now**. It's inside of you, and you don't need the assistance or permission of a cleric to access it.

Over the years, the masses were taught that God was separate from them. That belief caused people to give up their power to an unseen, fearful arbiter, or worse, to fallible, human "holy" men who could intercede for them because they were unworthy. The truth is this: You are the very incarnation of universal God consciousness here on Earth, and possess access to all the same creative power that brought you here, because you were created in the image and likeness of this power, and that means . . . you are as divine right now as you will ever be. To be God consciousness *is* to be divine. You could never be anything else.

We access this consciousness by going within, *not* without. When seeking answers, the Christian tradition tells us to be still and "enter into the secret place of the most high." This is a place in your consciousness, not on Earth. The same tradition tells us to "be *still* and know that I am God." It also says that we shall "be made whole by the *renewing of our minds*," and that the "meek shall inherit the earth". In many spiritual philosophies, earth is seen as a metaphor for the body. When we become still and go into the secret place of universal God consciousness, our body is rejuvenated and healing takes place.

MEDIA MADNESS

It's difficult to be still when we live in a world where everyone's attention is so fractured. Concentration has become a lost art in the age of cell phones, portable computers, internet-on-demand, iPods, texting, Blackberries, electronic books, instant messaging, Twitter, blogging, Facebook, video games, and Skype camera communication. As human beings, we're becoming more and more disengaged from one another. We're communicating more and saying less. **Remember that the most important thing you can ever give anyone or anything is your attention!** Living in the age of multitasking has taken its toll on our spiritual development. When you don't have the ability to focus for any length of time on any one thing, you diminish your capacity to connect to yourself and to universal God consciousness.

Researchers at Stanford University have shown that media multitaskers do not pay attention, control their memory, or switch from one job to another as well as those who perform one task at a time. They have much more difficulty filtering out irrelevant information and applying what they've learned when compared with those who are single-minded in their actions.[71] A study at the University of California at Los Angeles showed that media junkies actually *alter the structure and processes* by which their brains learn! Ordinarily, the hippocampus or section of the brain that's responsible for memory recall is active when we learn a singular new activity. When the attention of multitaskers gets divided, the hippocampus switches off, leading them to compensate with other areas of the brain and making information recall very difficult.[72]

Perhaps the saddest commentary on our media addiction comes from a recent *New York Times* poll that showed one in seven people admitted to spending less time with their spouses because of media gadgets, and one in ten said they spend less time with their children.[73] *The New York Times* also featured a profile of five college professors who ventured into Glen Canyon National Recreation Area in Utah for one week as a media detox experiment. David Strayer from the University of Utah summed up the importance of attention when he said, "Attention is the Holy Grail. Everything you're conscious of, everything you let in, everything you remember and forget depends on it."[74]

It's interesting that we are in the middle of what's commonly called the Information Age. Think about what that means. To possess information is to be in "form." To be inspired with an answer you've been seeking is to be in "spirit." Where would you rather put your attention?

TIME ON YOUR SIDE

We create everything in our existence and that includes time. The only moment that ever exists is the current one, NOW. In reality, there is no past or future, just a neverending succession of NOWs. All that exists is the endless expanse of universal God consciousness in a perpetual state of NOW, which contains within it the creative idea of every single object, outcome, and situation that could ever be contemplated. Some refer to this consciousness as the infinite field of possibilities where all the information to create anything coexists at once.

When we think a thought, we reach out into this ever-present energy field and choose an idea, image, or information that pertains to the current situation we happen to be in. This "thought" creates an action or event in an otherwise, ever-present NOW. As we *keep thinking*, we generate more thought/events. It's the space *between* these thoughts that generate the illusion of time.

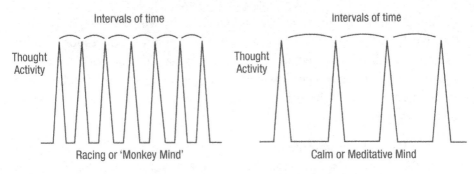

Thought/Time Correlation

Think of a hospital patient connected to a heart monitor. Every time his heart beats, it appears as a tall peak or spike on the screen. The spaces between beats, where the heart is resting, are seen as the low, straight-line valleys. Our thoughts are like these peaks. Time is the distance between them. The more thoughts we have in closer succession means *less* time between them. This is why when we are feeling rushed, frantic, out of time, or multitasking, time seems to move faster. *It literally does* because we're creating it that way. Every thought we think is a time/space event in an otherwise eternal NOW. The more thoughts we have, the faster our lives seem to fly by. When we consider the countless number of extraneous thoughts we generate every day, is it any wonder time seems to move faster as we get older and live less in the present moment?

On the contrary, a calm, meditative mind that remains in the present creates far fewer peaks or thought/events. Thus, the distance between them is much greater, creating fewer and longer spans of time. When we are relaxed and enjoying ourselves, time actually slows down as we get closer to the timeless state of NOW. As children, we had far fewer extraneous thoughts and worry habits. We weren't thinking all the time. We were simply enjoying NOW. That's why, as a child, a three-month summer vacation seemed twice as long. It was for us then, because we generated time at a completely different pace.

MAKING THE CONNECTION

Every answer we seek to any situation exists in universal God consciousness. The key to every physical, emotional, and spiritual healing is there waiting for us in *the gap between our thoughts*. To make this connection, we must get off our mental hamster wheels. Our intuition, higher Self, or divine guidance is constantly speaking to us, but it always speaks in a whisper. It is impossible to hear it above the level of mental noise most of us generate. The most powerful way to escape your "monkey mind" and connect with the infinite part of yourself that holds the answers you seek is through a regular practice of meditation.

There is no reason to be intimidated by meditation. It's simply an effective way to calm the mind. You don't need chanting, far Eastern symbols, or incense to make the connection. God consciousness is right where you are because it's *what* you are. Meditation is simply a calming practice to remove extraneous thoughts and create the mental space for the answers you seek to enter. I like to think that meditation simply turns the chattering monkey of my mind into a sacred "monk" with the "key" to the answers I need.

You're not trying to DO anything or reach any kind of specific "state." You're simply BEING in the moment. The best part is that while there are different styles of meditation, there is no wrong way to do it. Try this experiment. Close your eyes and say to yourself internally, *"I wonder what my next thought is going to be."* Do it now. What happened immediately after you asked yourself that question? **Nothing.** You simply waited in the open space between your thoughts. Congratulations! You just meditated.

Chances are, it only took a short time before an extraneous thought about your work or picking up dry cleaning broke the mental silence. The goal with meditation is to learn to go into that silent place for longer, uninterrupted periods of time. That space is where universal God consciousness speaks to us when we need guidance and answers about the big issues of our lives. When you take the time to ask, you will always get an answer. It may not come immediately, but I assure you, it will come. I cannot over-emphasize the healing power of meditation.

One Size Fits All

Meditation is not a religion. It's a mental discipline. Think of it as going to the gym for your mind. Virtually every religious belief system contains within it references to the power of meditation and the importance of connecting to universal God consciousness. So, it can easily compliment any spiritual belief system you currently adhere to.

As your practice, you'll notice that your ability to concentrate outside of your meditations will heighten considerably. This will help you stay much more attentive and focused on any task you're involved with. You'll experience an opening in your awareness where all the mental noise used to exist. Thought takes an extraordinary amount of energy. When you no longer have all those useless, compulsive, and habitual thoughts rambling around inside your mind, you'll have more mental and *physical* energy to devote to things that really matter to you. Your thought process will become faster and sharper. It's been said that the space shuttle uses 90% of its fuel just to break through Earth's atmosphere. Imagine how much fuel/energy we use when we're trapped in our monkey minds. When we breakout through that barrier, we regain an immeasurable amount of energy to consciously use as we desire. Since it literally slows down time, including your internal body clock, meditation also makes you look younger. How's that for a bonus?!

IN THE BEGINNING

When starting out, remember to not take meditation so seriously or you'll become frustrated and give up. It takes time and practice, just like any other new activity. Be dedicated, but not serious. The easiest thing to do is sit in a comfortable chair. Do not lie down or you're liable to fall asleep. Keep a watch or clock close by, and give yourself ten minutes. Take three deep breaths and exhale fully after each one. Close your eyes. Fold your hands in your lap and simply relax. Place your focus on your breath, particularly at the place where the air enters your nostrils. Just take note of each inhalation and exhalation. Don't try to change it if it's shallow or uneven. Just notice it. Keep your focus there for as long as you can. You might even say to yourself internally with each breath, "in," "out," and so on. Eventually, you'll be able to stop saying the words in your head and just be with your breath. At the start, however, this can be a helpful tool to keep you connected.

Irrelevant thoughts will break through—lots of them. The idea is not to prevent the thoughts from coming, but to *not engage* in any of them. As thoughts about work, the kids, or your favorite TV show come into view, simply let them float out of your mind like a cloud. Sometimes, they can come rapid-fire. Don't be discouraged. Just do your best to release them, and come back to the breath. There will be times when you're not even aware that you've been swept away by a thought until you've been entertaining it for several minutes. That's okay. When you do become aware, just come back to the breath.

Being a meditation beginner has a great benefit. You'll get a very clear picture of how rampant monkey mind can be. You'll discover that our minds aren't just filled with cluttered thoughts about current issues. Completely useless thoughts we're not even conscious of take up vital mental energy on a daily basis. During meditation, you might experience thoughts about a classmate you haven't seen since third grade, the possibility of UFOs existing, or how to make the best red velvet cake. You'll say to yourself, "Where did *that* come from?" Just let it go. It's just the layers of unnecessary mental clutter that have been siphoning off your attention and energy peeling away like the layers of an onion.

GOING DEEPER

As you continue, you may want to explore other types of meditation. Some use breath work, such as Vipassana meditation, while others like Japa, Vedic, and Transcendental meditation use mantras or the repetition of a specific word(s) to focus the mind. All of these techniques offer official training and most courses have nominal fees or are structured on a donation basis. It should be noted that Transcendental Meditation training can be quite expensive. The only reason for this is that it is taught by a foundation that requires business expenses to remain in operation. The other modes do not come with these costs. They have been handed down through thousands of years by an informal network of individual teachers who are not part of an official association and offer their services on a donation basis.

Once you've become comfortable with the basic technique described above, I would suggest that you explore Vedic meditation. It's a simple but powerful, mantra-based meditation technique very similar to Transcendental Meditation but without the high fees. You can find an instructor in your area at www.vedicnetwork.com. Vipassana meditation is also a great way to start a practice. Remember, your goal is simply to get into the gap between your thoughts and remain in that empty, peaceful place for longer periods of time. Ideally, you need to practice twice each day for just 10-15 minutes in the morning and at night. Eventually, you'll want to meditate twice a day for about 20-30 minutes each time. That's all. The effects of meditation are so powerful that you don't need to meditate for much longer than that. It's about quality, not quantity. Because you're retraining your mind and incorporating new muscle memory into you cells, you'll want to be consistent and use the same meditation space each time, if you can. Repetition and consistency are powerful accelerators in learning.

Be patient. The practice of meditation takes time but the rewards are beyond measure. I cannot express this enough. For me, the miracle of meditation is best described by U.S. Andersen in his groundbreaking book, *Three Magic Words*: "Everything proceeds from mind. Everything proceeds from thought and miracles are wrought in quiet hours in still rooms when awakened Souls harken their Divinity."[75]

Be Still, Go Within

I'm a disciple of love.
Don't talk about anything but sweetness, love and light
Yesterday I went completely crazy.
Love saw me.
"Don't wail. Don't tear your clothing.
I have come."
"Oh, Love," I cried out.
"I'm afraid of something else."
"Those other things don't even exist," he said.
"Be still and go within.
I'll whisper many secrets in your ear.
Just answer me by shaking your head.
Be still, go within."
"A moonlike soul has appeared
on the journey to the heart.
This journey to the heart is the most satisfying,
but stay still, go within."
This time I asked the heart,
"Oh heart, what kind of moon is that?"
He called back to me,
"This is not something that
you can understand with your mind.
Stay still, go within."
I persisted,
"Is this something angelic or human?"
"Neither," Love answered.
"Stay still, go within."
I said,
"I've just about passed out of myself
I feel turned completely upside down."

"Be like that,"
Heart said.
"Be still, so within."
"Oh one who stays in a house,
cluttered with shapes and images," Love said.
"Pack your belongings and get out of this place.
Just stay still and go into your heart."
"Oh, Heart," I begged.
"Please treat me paternalistically.
Isn't that one of God's attributes?"
"Yes," he said.
"Of course it is but even then,
with the soul of parenting you
stay still, go within."

—*Jelaluddin Rumi, Persian poet*

REALITY CHECK ... HEAD SPACE

✓ Every material object is made of the same substance (energy). It comes into being from a single source, universal mind or God consciousness.

✓ This consciousness is forever seeking expansion through an endless evolution of life experiences . . . including yours and mine!

✓ We are like computers, downloading information of our choice from the universal consciousness, which play out on our screens as the circumstances of our lives.

✓ It is impossible for God consciousness to be anything but complete. It is whole. That means it contains within it the answer to every problem you seek.

✓ Through meditation, you align your energy with universal God consciousness and have access to intuitive power that far exceeds your intellect.

✓ Connecting with universal God consciousness is what brings about all healing.

✓ Multitasking reduces our attention and our ability to connect to ourselves, each other, and God consciousness.

✓ The Information Age has left us hyper-focused on information and stuck in the illusion of form. To receive the answers we seek, we need to be inspired or in spirit.

✓ We create everything in our life experience, including time.

✓ Frantic, rambling thoughts make our lives move faster by speeding up time.

✓ A calm, meditative mind lengthens time because it's outside of it. It's in the NOW.

✓ Meditation allows us to quiet our inner voices so we can hear the voice of God.

✓ Like life, connecting with universal God consciousness is simple. It couldn't be easier because it's right where you are and it's *what* you are.

✓ Meditation has no religious affiliation but can complement any faith you subscribe to.

✓ Meditate for 15-20 minutes twice each day. Use the same space for consistency.

FOOD FOR THOUGHT

Task Master

This exercise is one of the simplest, yet most challenging, you'll find in this book. It's simple because there's nothing special you need to do. It's difficult because we've trained ourselves to live in a completely different way.

Choose a day that you know isn't going to be terribly hectic. That probably means a day where you're not working. So, a weekend or holiday off from your job might be ideal. During the entire day, *do NOT multitask*. Perform **only one** task at a time. If you're watching TV, eating chips, and polishing your nails, you're performing three tasks simultaneously. Talking on the phone while checking email is two tasks. Driving, listening to music, and eating a sandwich is three tasks. If you're eating, just eat. If you're reading, just read. If you're on the phone, just talk on the phone while doing nothing else.

You'll be surprised how difficult it is to sustain this kind of focus for a full 24-hour period. You'll come to understand why some people can have a tough time at the outset trying to get a meditation practice going. You'll see how you continue to feed your monkey mind. Eventually, you'll regain control of your attention. I highly recommend continuing with this when and where you can and you'll find that as it becomes easier to direct your focus, the activities themselves will become their own meditation. That's why activities like gardening can be so relaxing. When we do them with a singular focus, they actually become meditations for us. The Eastern cultures have known this for millennia and even practice walking meditations.

CHAPTER 12

THE RHYTHM OF LIFE
EXPANSION & CONTRACTION

"The best way out is always though."

—Robert Frost, *poet*

"Even the darkness of the soil provides nourishment for the seed."

—Anonymous

"But I say unto you, they [joy and sorrow] are inseparable.
Together they come and when one sits alone with you
at your board, remember that the other is asleep upon your bed."

—Kahlil Gibran, *author*

Whenever life seems to make no sense (and remember, it makes *perfect* sense), I always look to nature to remind myself of how deceptively simple it really is. Life is about creating balance through a continuous cycle of renewal. We see the signs of balance everywhere, from the tides to the seasons. Still, we seem to miss the idea of what is actually required for renewal to take place. Renewal means *new* growth. Something *new* is created. To create something new, space must be made for its arrival, hence the phrase, "out with the old and in with the new." That means that whatever currently exists must pass away for the new to enter. The leaves of autumn must die before the buds of spring can blossom. Lightning must strike the Great Plains and create wildfires to clear out the dead brush before the pastures can be green again.

A volcano violently purges the lava that ultimately increases the land mass of its island.

This system of natural balance is obvious to us when we look at things like summer and winter, day and night, or life and death. It's everywhere. Because we are in the world and made of the exact same energy as everything that surrounds us, why is it so hard to understand that our lives were designed to ebb and flow to this very same rhythm?

BALANCE OF OPPOSITES

All things that appear of opposite nature to us are really two sides of the same coin. What appears to us as "good" or "bad" really serves the same purpose. Is the sun any more important than the rain in the growth of a tree? No. They're both equally important. If a tree were only exposed to the sun and no rain, or vice versa, it would quickly die. The darkness of the soil is just as vital to the nourishment of a seed as the sunlight that will eventually feed it. This alternating dance between light and dark is what creates the process we call life. The ancients knew this and celebrated the dark side of life as well as the light, knowing that one was equally dependent on the other. This understanding is most notably expressed in the Yin Yang symbol of Taoism. In this symbol, the dark and light sides of life fit together perfectly in a never-ending circle.

I like to think of this balance of opposites as the Law of Expansion and Contraction. This divine process of renewal not only rules over nature, but our lives, as well. Because everything is made of exactly the same vibrating energy, it means that every single object in life is always in some state of expansion or contraction. Remember those invisible energy "strings" that we learned about earlier? It's like having a piece of poster board in your hands and shaking it so that it bows outward into a convex shape and backward into a concave shape trillions of times per second. Yes, the very energy of your body obeys the Law of Expansion and Contraction. Expansion and contraction is the rhythm of life. Your heart is doing it about 75 times per minute, and that's what keeps you alive. Nothing stands still. We live in a universe of constant motion. Even a rock in your backyard is moving because the energy within it is in a constant state of expansion and contraction, even though you can't see it.

DISTORTING THE DANCE

As human beings, we experience expansion and contraction in our lives as joy and sorrow. If we get a raise at work, we feel fantastic and we're in a state of expansion. When we get a serious diagnosis from the doctor, we become fearful and sad as we enter a state of contraction. The difficulty in managing our lives comes when we forget that life is really the balance of opposites. We judge circumstances as either good *or* bad. We end up becoming addicted to situations that provide us with expansion and fear those where we'll experience contraction. We've distorted the dance of life and fallen out of the natural flow.

Because we fear contraction is something bad, we avoid or resist it. As a result, we send out more fearful energy, bringing back to us more fear and contraction by way of the Law of Attraction. What we resist persists. We've forgotten that our troubles are equally essential to our growth as our triumphs. Unfortunately, we see them as nuisances or delays in our life progress brought on by some external person or circumstance. We just don't have time for problems! We may think contraction stalls our life progress, but nothing could be further from the truth. The movement of life isn't in either expansion or contraction, but in *the momentum generated between the two* as they constantly trade places in our lives. The key to moving forward is to not resist either state when it comes to visit us, but to willingly and fully go into the experience. Like a child on a swing, we know that the deeper we lean backward into that position, the stronger and faster our forward momentum will be *out of* that position. When we resist our contraction, we stop the natural momentum of our lives, and we literally become stuck in a particular situation. How many times have you felt stuck in your life? Those are the times you've been resisting the natural flow of expansion and contraction.

A caterpillar has the rhythm of life completely figured out. If he were to stay in a constant state of expansion, he'd be an inert blob sprawled out on the sidewalk. If he were to stay in a constant state of contraction, he'd be curled up into a ball going nowhere. Instead, he uses the rhythm generated between the states of expansion and contraction to propel himself forward and get where he wants to go. He knows his bodily contractions are just as important as his expansions in moving him forward. If he saw his contractions as problems or setbacks and kept trying to avoid them, he'd be stuck, too, and probably end up as lunch for a blackbird.

It's by working in cooperation between these two different states of being that the caterpillar accomplishes his goal: simply to travel a great distance to a high tree branch and create a cocoon. By working *with* his expansions and contractions, he has led himself to his destination that will provide for his complete metamorphosis. It's easy to think when we're in the middle of a contraction that we'll never make it out, but there's a wonderful anonymous saying that goes, "Just when the caterpillar thought the world was over, he turned into a butterfly."

EXPANSION ADDICTION

When we experience contraction, we usually react in one of two ways. Many of us jump into our "doing" mode to get rid of the problem. Doing only leads us into frustration because it's a resistant action that tries to attack and eradicate the problem by focusing on . . . the problem. It's a masculine, yang energy: the doer, warrior, analyst. The problem with this approach is that healing, which is an expansive experience, comes from BEING, not doing. Expansion is feminine or yin energy: the healer, moderator, nurturer. To properly heal, we must develop our yin energy. Many of the world's problems today come from the expression of too much yang energy.

On the other hand, we can create artificial expansion for ourselves to avoid the pain of contraction. This is the heart of all addiction. We do it through food, sex, drugs, shopping, alcohol, or even "busy-itis"—intentionally keeping ourselves so busy we can't possibly focus on what's really bothering us. The problem with this approach comes as we try desperately to hang onto our periods of false expansion for longer and longer periods of time. As we resist the natural cycle and try to cling to expansion, we generate a huge amount of fear and stress which are feelings of contraction, defeating our purpose. At the same time, our intuitive voice that guides us toward healing tells us this forced expansion is not really nurturing at all.

We avoid contraction and seek out expansion because it's what we were taught. For the first few years of our lives, we lived in the natural flow of opposites, crying/laughing, sleeping/waking, and so on. At some point, we're told to stop crying, whining, or throwing a temper tantrum. Suddenly, it's NOT okay to express how we feel. We come to learn that contractive emotions are bad, painful, and carry terrible consequences. We must avoid them at all costs. Worse yet, we learn that as we adapt to these new demands we earn our parents' approval. To a child, approval and love are the same thing. Without our parents' love and approval, who would take care of us? We would surely die. So, avoiding contraction becomes a way of survival for us. We'll do anything to accomplish it. It's the beginning of denying ourselves to please others. It's the moment we cease to be human *beings*. All the second-guessing, overcompensating, pandering, and self-censoring changes us into human *doings*. Is it any wonder why we avoid contraction so fiercely? Subconsciously, we still feel we will actually die if we go deep enough into the experience to discover what it's trying to tell us.

SAYING YES

When we have problems with our bodies through weight gain or even disease, we tend to think they've broken down, failed us or that there is something wrong with them. On the contrary, we have these problems because our bodies are working perfectly. These "problems" are the outward signal that something deeper is going on and we need to look within for the cause. Many people have said that their experience with cancer, heart disease, or other ailments was one of the best things to happen to them, not because of the associated physical pain, but because of how their lives changed as a result of the event. They chose to say YES to the opportunity to investigate the negative beliefs or energy their outward conditions were mirroring. They saw the *purpose* in their problem and, thus, didn't focus on the problem itself. It was their wake-up call to heal relationships, practice forgiveness, or give love that would greatly improve the quality of their lives. We all have pain, but we can eliminate the suffering associated with it if we choose to see the purpose in it. Many faiths teach that to experience pain without suffering is a noble truth.

This is why more physicians are learning to address adverse physical conditions such as obesity or cancer as disease. As scary as these situations might seem, they're really the body's way of talking to us, telling us we're living in a body/mind that is not "at ease." When we say we have a particular disease, it implies there is some foreign element attacking us and immediately sets up an adversarial relationship. When we see our state of disease as a messenger with our call to return to wholeness, we recognize it as our ally and say YES to the situation as it is.

When we choose to fight our situation by going on another diet or just treating our symptoms, we're shooting the messenger. We're telling our body that we don't trust it. When we say NO to its opportunity to heal, we're saying YES to disease. Remember, the universe is an *affirmative* place. It's always saying YES, and so should you . . . to the contraction that's guiding you inward to where your real healing resides.

PUSH OR PULL

Early in my career, I ran an integrative medical clinic in downtown Los Angeles. During that time, I treated a large number of patients with dog bites, mostly postal carriers. Treating a dog bite is complicated. The flesh tears are usually very uneven, so doctors don't suture them. This gives the wound the ability to heal from the inside out and avoid infection. Basically, the wound is left open. After a few years, I noticed there were only two types of patients: those who healed beautifully and effortlessly from their wounds, and those who did not. A brief study in canine anatomy brought me the answer.

A dog's teeth are angled backwards toward the rear of the mouth. It's the perfect design for gripping and ripping meat. If your hand happens to be in the jaws of a dog, the worst thing you can do is try to pull away. This action only drives the reverse-angle teeth further into the flesh, resulting in a more severe injury. Counter-intuitive as it seems, the best thing to do is push the hand further *into* the dog's mouth. This activates its gag reflex and it releases the hand.

A martial arts principle states, "Push when pulled and pull when pushed." It teaches us not to use force in defending against a forceful action. The best strategy is to use the opponent's own energy against him. When he approaches with a pushing motion, the rival is to grab his forward-moving hand or foot and pull him to the ground, using his own energy, force, and intention.

Unlike a boxer, whose stance is closed and protected, a martial artist remains open and relaxed, inviting his challenger. If we are to heal our lives, we must remain open to receive all life has for us, including the challenges. The key is to stay out of "reaction" mode and channel the energy of the situation into our discovery of what it's there to teach us. It means to stay conscious and become a partner with the problem instead of its opponent. As we learn the lesson and move to a higher level of consciousness, the "teacher" passes and we move on. When we pull away from life's contractions, it only guarantees us a deeper wound, slower healing process, and messier scar.

Good Times and the Dark Side

Going within sometimes brings up memories or unconscious feelings that can be scary. You might say, *"But I thought I was supposed to focus on feeling good."* The goal in healing is to stop being manipulated by outer circumstances and to enter your experiences of contraction consciously and willingly. The idea is to open your emotional channels back up that were shut down earlier in life. When those channels are opened, the unexpressed and repressed energy can be released and healing energy can flow freely through you again. The intention is not to feel bad, but to remain open to any feelings that come to the surface and allow them to be consciously and completely experienced. We're not here to deny our feelings. That results in disease. Neither are we here to cry or rage on in self-proclaimed victimhood for years on end. Cooperating with our contraction means becoming conscious of WHAT we feel, WHEN we're feeling it, and WHY we're feeling it. Only then can our emotions be properly and completely discharged from our emotional and physical bodies. Then, we can make a *conscious* choice as to how we'd like to feel.

Sometimes, healing and contractive emotions can be very dark. Most of us don't want to admit that we have a dark side, or refuse to go there because it scares us. Too often we don't express our hurts and dishonor ourselves by brushing our feelings under the carpet of *"Oh, that's okay."* We pride ourselves on being "easy-going" and "rolling with the punches." We consider ourselves too "spiritually enlightened" to be upset about anything until all that repressed energy finds its own way out . . . in a BIG way. We dishonor our emotions when we engage in this kind of psycho-spiritual bypass. There's an old saying that goes, "Beware the anger of a quiet man."

When we deny our feelings long enough, we move away from our balance of opposites. We become disconnected from our bodies and intuition. We can enter a gray zone where we don't feel much at all. We're frustrated, bored, depressed, irritable, or apathetic. All of these emotions are masking something much deeper. When we can feel our emotions fully at the moment we experience them, we effectively discharge the negative energy and reset ourselves back on a positive track. We can avoid the gray zone where so many people meander through lives half-lived.

EMOTIONAL ANTI-VENOM

One of the pain interventions I offer in my practice is known as apitherapy, or bee venom therapy. It dates back to the 1930s and is very simple. When a bee injects venom into its victim, blood immediately rushes to the area, flooding it with oxygen and healing compounds. In a controlled process, patients receive actual bee stings in their problem areas. As a byproduct, the injury in that area receives the same benefit from the oxygen-rich blood rush. Patient improvements are often dramatic. I believe this therapy is very healing in these cases, but there is another factor at play. Pain is often equated with repressed anger. In this case, the angry bee injects not only its venom into the patient, but its intention of anger, as well. In this way, the bee's venom (anger) acts like an emotional homeopathic anti-venom for the patient's unexpressed anger.

So often we fear our dark emotions like shame, guilt, or regret. We fear that if we stay open to our contraction, the emotion will destroy us. So we close down to protect ourselves. Actually, the opposite is true. Repressed negative emotions create some of the most poisonous and disease-causing cytokines in the body, far more toxic than any venom. To release painful emotions, we must allow ourselves to fully experience them. Pain is its own anti-venom. Emotional awareness is the antidote to self-intoxication. The *Gnostic Gospels* of the Dead Sea Scrolls are quite direct in emphasizing the importance of clearing our emotional house.

> *"If you bring forth what is within you, what you bring forth will save you. If you do not bring forth what is within you, what you do not bring forth will destroy you."*—**Jesus Christ**, Gospel of St. Thomas

When we say YES to our contraction, we fully release stagnant energy from our hearts. The Universe hates a void. It **must** be filled with something. When you clear up space in your heart for love to enter, miracles happen.

I had been working with a patient recently who was diagnosed with prostate cancer. In addition to the physical treatment I was providing, I assisted the patient in exploring what emotional issues might be contributing to his situation. After some time, he was comfortable enough to share with me that for many years, he'd felt like a failure as a husband and father. As he recalled all the times he felt he'd made bad choices, all his grief, sadness, regret, and shame came flooding to the surface. He must have felt very safe with me, because he gave himself permission to feel all of these emotions in full as he wept for his past mistakes. It took nearly an hour before he could catch his breath. Afterward, he confided in me that he'd never shared these things with anyone, *ever*.

When he returned to his home country, he made his scheduled visit with his regular physician. After several weeks, he called me. He was very excited and said his doctor told him, "I don't know what you've been doing in California, but keep doing it. Your current tests show no sign of cancer."

I don't know if I believe in magic bullets, but I do believe in brave patients. It took an extreme amount of bravery for this man to willingly go that deeply into his contraction. It's no coincidence that he felt emasculated for so many years and that his cancer showed up in the master male gland. Instinctively, he knew that the cancer wasn't his problem, but how he was relating to it. To fully discharge his pain, he took a very big emotional risk, and as a result, created a void where healing moved in . . . in an equally big way.

Act II

Recently, I took a trip to the Middle East and had gone to visit an ancient church. It didn't seem like my tour group was in the right location, because we were led up to the front of what appeared to be an impenetrable, rocky mountainside. How could there possibly be a church here? Then, I was directed to enter the mountain through a tiny hole cut into its exterior. The crude opening couldn't have been more than four feet high. It wasn't a comfortable experience to crouch down far enough to fit through the cramped space. Once I did, I couldn't believe what I saw. This tiny hole opened up to one of the tallest, most beautiful sanctuaries I'd ever seen. There was no possible way to even imagine the beauty that lay hidden inside this gigantic rock without shrinking down and passing through the cramped opening. It was then that I was reminded of the importance of contraction and expansion in our lives.

Science uses the term *liminality* to describe it. It means to be on a threshold, in a passageway between two worlds. That experience reminded me of the necessity to accept a brief moment of discomfort or contraction, and that if I cooperated with it I would pass through into a new expansion. *Every contraction in life is setting you up for another expansion.* It MUST. *That is the rhythm of life.* The sooner we flow into the experience, the quicker our next expansion will arrive. It's like watching a stage play. The curtain always has to fall *before* the next act can begin.

Expansion in the Body

Healing exists in expansion, but most people don't fully understand it. They mistake expansion as a state of happiness based on owning physical possessions or when circumstances go their way. True expansion is an openness, an awareness in which we are completely exposed, vulnerable, and available to accept life just as it is in this moment, with an open heart. It is in that moment, when our heart is fully open—or broken open as some might say—that love and healing have the space to move in.

Making love is a great example of expansion and contraction. The initial stages are mostly contractive experiences leading up to orgasm. Most people would mistake orgasm as the expansion, but it's not. It's extreme contraction. Expansion happens in the moments immediately *afterward*, when the partners and the experience all seem to merge into one entity. There is no I, you, or me anymore. It's the moment of surrender, a place of total release where we collapse into absolute being. It's a remembering of our wholeness.

Our society has come to worship the orgasm as the destination of sex, but it's only the *doorway* to a fuller, truer experience. This kind of surrender is so complete that it terrifies most people. That's why they'd rather roll over and go to sleep immediately after orgasm and return to unconsciousness.

On the physical plain, expansion is also like the feeling you get after a strenuous workout. You're exhausted because of what you've just been through, but you're energized and feel stronger at the same time. Expansion is a state of BEING after the constant "doing" or resisting is done. This is why so many of us reach a place of expansion only *after* we've tried everything we know of to solve our problem. We hit our rock bottom and have a breakdown-or-breakthrough moment. It's in *that place* of pure beauty and fragility that healing finally arrives.

BRING IT ON

A lot of people think that accepting a moment of contraction is the same as quitting, throwing in the towel. It's giving power to the fat, disease, or problem. It's not. When you scramble from diet to diet or from one miracle cure to another; you're giving your power away to fear. It's resistance. When we surrender to what is, just in this moment . . . not forever. We take our power back. We summon our courage, go within for our answers, and say, "Bring it on. I can handle this." We get out of the fear of DOING and open space for receiving. From that perspective, we finally see that expansion and contraction have their source in the same light. They are like our favorite and hardest teachers in high school. It's only when we look back from a more mature perspective that we can appreciate the invaluable lessons they *both* taught us.

THE GUEST HOUSE

This being human is a guest house.
Every morning a new arrival.

A joy, a depression, a meanness,
some momentary awareness comes
as an unexpected visitor.

Welcome and entertain them all!
Even if they are a crowd of sorrows,
who violently sweep your house
empty of its furniture,
still, treat each guest honorably.
He may be clearing you out
for some new delight.

The dark thought, the shame, the malice.
meet them at the door laughing and invite them in.

Be grateful for whatever comes.
because each has been sent
as a guide from beyond.

— *Jelaluddin Rumi*, *Persian poet*

Reality Check ... The Rhythm of Life

✓ The renewal of life is governed by the Law of Expansion & Contraction.

✓ We experience expansion as positive experiences and contraction as negative ones.

✓ The momentum of life is generated as expansion and contraction trade places in our lives.

✓ When we resist our contraction, we stop life's momentum and we become stuck.

✓ Healing is an expansive experience; a feminine BEING energy—not doing.

✓ Creating artificial expansion to avoid our contractions results in addictive behavior.

✓ Saying YES to your contraction means being willing to discover what the problem is trying to teach us, *rather than the problem itself.*

✓ When we see our problem as a call to return to wholeness, it becomes our ally, and we say YES to the situation as it is, reducing resistance.

✓ The universe is AFFIRMATIVE. When we fight our contraction through constant dieting or symptom management, we're telling the universe we want to continue fighting.

✓ When we learn the lesson of any contraction, the "teacher" moves on from our lives.

✓ Cooperating with our contraction means becoming conscious of WHAT we feel, WHEN we're feeling it, and WHY we're feeling it.

✓ Feeling our emotions fully in each moment discharges negative energy and keeps the momentum of expansion and contraction moving through our lives.

✓ Negative emotions are their own antidote when we can feel them completely.

✓ When we surrender to what is in the moment, we take our power back from the fear of "DOING" and we make space for receiving.

✓ **Every contraction in life is setting you up for another expansion.** It MUST. That is the rhythm of life.

FOOD FOR THOUGHT

Invisible Expansion

Because we judge all of our experiences as good or bad, we're unaware of the good things the process of expansion and contraction has brought us in our lives. Perhaps a relationship you had that ended badly was more than a heartbreaking contraction. Maybe the expansion was learning to stand on your own two "financial" feet and a well-earned sense of independence. Take some time to list the biggest moments of contraction in your life. Looking back on them now, how were you changed by the experiences in a positive way? What was the expansion you experienced after passing through those temporary moments of discomfort? What type of expansion might the situation with your weight or health now be leading you to?

Contraction	*Expansion*

CHAPTER 13

THE PILLARS OF PERSONAL CHANGE

I. SELF-LOVE

*"You can search throughout the entire universe for someone
who is more deserving of your love and affection than you are yourself,
and that person is not to be found anywhere. You yourself as much
as anybody in the entire universe deserve your love and affection."*

—Buddha

*"Love creates, produces, heals, comforts, guides, illumines.
He who makes himself one with love makes himself one with God,
and God works through him."*

—U.S. Andersen, *author*

*"Love is an element, though physically unseen, is as
real as air or water. It is an acting, living, moving force."*

—Prentice Mulford, *author*

In some languages, there are as many as 50 different words to express the idea of love. In English, we have **one**. Is it any wonder that there is so much confusion when it comes to understanding love and the role it plays in healing and transformation? We know that becoming aware of how our beliefs, thoughts and feelings interact with our bodies energetically is a powerful tool for changing our lives. As potent as these universal principles are, you cannot begin to use them consciously in any significant way unless they're supported by what I call the three **Pillars of Personal Change: Self-Love, Self-Acceptance, and Self-Forgiveness.**

BACK TO YOU

Self-love is far more than just doing something nice for yourself. In psychotherapy, we're often encouraged to buy that dress we've always wanted, take an overdue vacation, or set aside personal time as ways to love ourselves. In truth, these *are* loving actions we take toward ourselves, but they don't generate much feeling or lasting emotion. Remember that how we feel in any one moment is the key to creating change. Love is the most powerful force in the universe and the highest feeling frequency we can experience. Love is not a sentimental notion. It is a **real, dynamic, and measurable scientific energy**. We've already seen that the Institute of HeartMath has proven that the electromagnetic field of the heart is 5,000 times stronger than that of the brain. In an additional study, it's been shown that when two people touch in a loving way, one person's electrocardiogram (ECG) signal *actually registers* in the other person's electroencephalogram (EEG) and in other areas of their body. The two people don't even have to be touching for this exchange to occur. They need only be in close proximity. This has proven that when we are loving to others, a real exchange of bioelectrical heart energy is transferred between individuals.[76]

So how do we love ourselves? What does that really mean? It seems so simple, yet difficult at the same time. Love does not exist in a vacuum. We live in an orderly, dynamic universe governed by laws, including the Law of Attraction. Like a divine game of pitch-and-catch, this scientific principle tells us that whatever we seek we must give *first* in order for it to return to us. Understanding this, we can see that loving others IS loving yourself, because in doing so, all that love must return to you. By this divine order, it's our relationships that heal us.

A Persian parable tells the story of a man who died and found himself in a beautiful meadow filled with the most luscious fruit trees and abundant foods he'd ever seen. Even so, everyone there appeared grossly underweight and visibly malnourished. He asked where he was, and a passerby told him he was in hell. He couldn't understand the condition of the inhabitants of this place until he saw them sit down to eat. Everyone had locked elbow joints.

Even though they were surrounded by the most delicious foods, no one could reach their own mouth to eat it. Shortly thereafter, he found himself in an identical meadow teeming with ripe foods. A man welcomed him to heaven. He was completely confused because the meadow looked exactly the same, but the people here looked beautiful and robust. The answer became evident when he saw the group sit down to eat. Although their elbows were also locked, they reached across the table and fed each other.

Getting It Out

Psychotherapy can be a wonderful tool for helping us discover the roots of our negative patterns. Once we discover them however, we can become stuck in the idea that we have to "get it all out" in regard to our anger, rage, jealousy, sadness, loneliness or other destructive emotions. We've seen how essential it is to recognize, honor and release our negative emotions and energy. All healing requires it. The problem occurs when we're still "releasing" these emotions years later, waiting for a specific moment when we know it's "all gone." To me, there is a distinct difference between properly releasing a negative emotion, and continually re-traumatizing yourself by reliving a bad experience over and over again. Even if you do get to a point where you feel you may have "gotten it all out," what then? You're still left with a void. What fills that space in your heart?

When it comes to love, most people's hearts are like a glass half-full of water. They're only half-full of love or less! We spend far too many years trying to figure out what's "wrong" with us, trying to get all the anger, fear, sadness, rage, and pain out of our hearts. You can't fill the glass up by fighting the emptiness. *The emptiness disappears when you pour more love in.* You put love in by extending your love to others, knowing it will return to you and fill you back up. Don't worry so much about the darkness. The darkness automatically goes when the light is turned on.

All There Is

Love is the master law of the universe. Love *is* the Law of Attraction. Why do you want anything you want in your life? You want it because you *love* it. You love how you'll look in your ideal body so you're changing your lifestyle. You love Italian food, so you go to that kind of restaurant. You love a particular kind of car, so you're saving to buy one. Love is the creative power of life. It generates our desires and dreams.

Think back on your most loving memories. Maybe it was the birth of a child or the success of helping a friend achieve a hard-won goal. You can't feel any better than when you're giving and receiving love like that. Because these moments are super-charged with feelings of love and self-love as a result; you are attracting all the things you love to you at warp speed. It doesn't matter if its weight loss, more income, a better relationship or health. They're all being drawn to you as long as you remain in a place of loving. That's why it's always the "magnetic" person who is so gregarious and loving that seems to have everything going his way. He's attracting all the things he loves to him by being free with his own loving.

No Lack

We know all that really exists is energy, waiting to be directed into form by our thoughts and desires. Where do our desires come from? They're born out of our love for something. So at its very core, we have a universe governed by love. Love is all there is. The universe is like a loving parent, willing to give us anything we choose by making all possibilities and potentialities available to us. All we have to do is ask consistently with our thoughts and feelings. Sure, we stumble, make mistakes and create things we don't intend while trying to use this amazing gift, but even our missteps are blessings in disguise. A child will never learn to ride a bicycle if the parent is constantly steadying it for him. He only learns about balance by falling down.

Love is the only creative, energetic force in existence. What were you told about energy in grade school science class? Energy has no beginning and no end. It always was and will be. It cannot be created or destroyed. What have all the ancient sages told us about God? God always was and will be. God has no beginning and no end. God cannot be created or destroyed. Understanding this, we can clearly see that *God is love moving according to divine universal laws in a never-ending process of creation.* All those bumper stickers from the 1970s were right. God *is* love. The holy texts tell us that "He who hasn't loved hasn't known God, for God is love." That's why when we live our lives from a place of love, the power of creation moves through us manifesting changes we could only otherwise describe as miracles.

Love is the ultimate, divine law. Love is all there is. If that's so, then it's impossible for it to have an "opposite." What about the world's problems, you say? Where is the love in war, poverty and disease? Those things are nothing but a lack of peace, abundance and health, which are all products of love. The world's problems exist because of a lack of love, not a lack of food, money or other resources. When you choose to step into your loving, there will be no lack in your life, either.

LOVE HEALS

If God *is* love and nothing imperfect can exist in the presence of God; then healing is simply the process of bringing love to the places within us that are hurting. Too many of us want to rush to a wonder drug or super herb to heal our bodies when what we're really crying out for is love. We do this, not so much as a search for a "quick fix," but as an unconscious way of avoiding what scares us most: the courage to release our pain and the vulnerability to allow love to enter. We're afraid to risk being hurt again because of how we were treated in the past. When we close ourselves off and don't give our love, we stop the flow of love's healing, creative energy from moving through us.

Human cells in a lab dish can only move in two directions; forward into growth or backward into protection. They will expand or move toward nourishment or contract and move away from toxins. They cannot do both as the same time. They must choose. If you remain in a state of negative emotion such as fear, anger, depression or stress, you're creating a tidal wave of toxic cytokines in your bloodstream. As a result, your cells contract, pull away from these dangerous elements and **stop growing**. By the principle of expansion and contraction, everything in life is either actively growing or dying. There is no in-between. The more "protection" you think you need, the more you shut off your growth/healing mechanism! When you're in the midst of a "fight-or-flight" response, the last thing your body is worried about is growth and healing. It's setting you up to run away from danger. In short, the less you love, the faster you die. The key to all healing, whether emotional or physical is the courage to love.

Research done at the Institute of HeartMath has proven what we've known intuitively about love's effect on the body. Specially trained test subjects were given samples of DNA in test tubes and instructed to generate intense feelings of love while holding the specimens. In less than two minutes, the DNA samples stretched out, opened up and expanded in significant ways. When the subjects expressed feelings of anger, hatred or frustration, the DNA constricted, shrank down and even switched off many genes! Amazingly, the subjects were separated from their samples and told to direct their emotions at the specimens from a different location. The same response occurred, completely independent of time and space. The experiment was ended when the subjects were a half mile away from the samples, with the same results.[77] This speaks volumes to the healing power of love right down to our DNA. It's become quite clear that the root of all weight gain and disease processes lies in our emotional states. The extent to which we're open to love conditions our genetic expression from moment to moment.

TWO CHOICES

When it comes right down to it, there are really only two emotions we can experience: love and the lack of love, which is fear. Fear is the father of all negative emotions including hate, anger and resentment. Just like our cells, we are being presented with a choice every minute of every day: love or fear. It doesn't matter what situation we find ourselves in or how badly someone has upset us. We can choose to ground ourselves in our loving or react out of fear. The choice is ours and our bodies are listening. No matter where I find myself or in what situation, I always ask before I act: *Where is the love in this?* If I can't answer that question, I choose a different response. The amount of growth you experience in your life will always be directly proportionate to the amount of love or fear you give. Once you truly understand that you and your neighbor are ONE on an energetic and spiritual level, it's so much easier to remain in a place of love. You won't be inclined to take an unloving action against him because to do so would be acting against yourself. Being grounded in loving means taking all action from an understanding of ONENESS.

LOVE KNOT

The problem for most of us in Western society is that we confuse real love with romantic love. We are all ONE within the great love that is God. We are made in the image and likeness of God and therefore *we are love itself*. It is the very fabric of our being. We only appear separate, living in different bodies

Life Growth Ratio

$$\text{Growth} = \frac{Love}{Fear}$$

seeking out individual adventures in this life. Intuitively, we have a drive to return to the oneness of God and end the illusion of separation. That's why we seek out relationships and why humans gravitate toward each other in a myriad of different groups. It's much more than simple friendship, common interests, or even romance. It's our drive to return to oneness, our true nature of pure love. These relationships, particularly romantic associations, are the closest we can ever come to a physical unification with God in this life. If we become conscious of why we seek out these kinds of relationships, we can allow ourselves to be healed by them instead of falling into possessiveness, insecurity, and petty jealousy. An intimate, loving relationship isn't about Hollywood. It's about wholeness.

Sex within intimate relationships is akin to real love as it's a situation where we seek to give and receive pleasure. A healthy sex life free of judgments, shame, and old wives' tales is one of the purest forms of loving expression. Historical rhetoric and dogma have only intended to separate us from our true nature by demoralizing our innate desire to return to ONENESS. If you want to examine your understanding of love and the healing power of relationships, you need look no further than the quality of your current intimate relationship.

TWO-WAY STREET

Whether romantic or platonic, it's important to remember that love in any kind of relationship is always a two-way street. It can be easy for someone to give love, but nearly impossible for them to accept a kind word or gesture from someone else. These folks become unintentional martyrs as they say, *"No thank you. I'll do without,"* or, *"That's okay. You really didn't need to do that for me."* Be aware that when love comes to you, you must accept it! If you do not, you are rejecting love and stopping the natural flow of it in your life. Freely accept kindness, offerings, and help knowing that this is YOUR love coming back to you. Say, *"Thank you,"* return the love, and keep the flow going! If you're a martyr personality, you may need to look at your beliefs about deservingness.

On the flipside, some people are great at accepting kindness from others. They're great "takers," but never give anything back. They feel love makes them weak. Remember that love never allows someone to take advantage of you. If it doesn't feel good, it's not love. Sometimes the most loving decision you can make for yourself and someone else is to say, "No."

OPEN TO LOVE

Real love is a state of BEING, not doing. It is a passive state that requires you to do nothing but recognize that *you are it* and allow it to flow through you to others. If you make the choice to step into love and away from fear in each moment of your life, you won't have to worry about monitoring all your beliefs, thoughts, and feelings. Actually, it's not possible to monitor every single one of them. When you think, act, and speak from love, you will be operating from a place where it is impossible for negativity to exist. As you do this, your body and life circumstances will begin to realign immediately, because the power of love *is* the power that heals.

II. SELF-ACCEPTANCE

"Nothing is a greater impediment to being on good terms with others than being ill at ease with yourself."

—Honore de Balzac, *French novelist*

"There is always a certain peace in being what one is, in being that completely."

—Ugo Betti, *Italian judge and author*

"It doesn't matter what we do until we accept ourselves. Once we accept ourselves, it doesn't matter what we do."

—Charly Heavenrich, *photographer*

It's not possible to love someone or something if we haven't accepted it. Without acceptance, there is only resistance. To truly love ourselves and others means to come from a place of non-judgment. It means to see situations as neither good nor bad, but simply as what is in this moment. It means to see people, beginning with ourselves, not as we wish they were, but as they are, and allow them to be exactly that. We're so hard on ourselves most of the time. We see ourselves as unattractive, lazy, untalented, undisciplined, stupid, selfish, or a failure. Would you love anyone with these qualities? Then how could you possibly expect to love yourself, or anyone else to love you, if you judge yourself this way?

I'm Okay, You're Okay

You might say that you're willing to accept the fact that you haven't been successful at relationships or bad with money but it's just impossible to accept your current weight. As long as there is even **one issue** about you or your life that you regret or resent, it will be impossible to achieve true self-acceptance. You are a complete soul. How can you accept only part of something that is whole? You must either take it fully or leave it completely. Self-acceptance is NOT conditional. It means accepting all of ourselves and allowing it to be okay right now. Just as we are. Just right now. Not forever. It won't last forever. Nothing does. It's just the way it is now, so we agree not to resist it. Resisting any situation is to fight it and apply force. As a result, we're met with an equal counterforce from the universe, and the situation *will* persist as long as we refuse to accept it as part of our present circumstance. Notice I didn't say part of yourself . . . but just as part of your present circumstance. As a Spiritual Soul, you are eternal, but circumstances are only temporary.

Our pets love us unconditionally. Because they are conscious but not "self-conscious," it's impossible for them to judge. They do not see us through the warped lens of our self-perceptions. They see us as courageous protectors and loving providers. They see in us all the qualities that really matter. What difference does it make to them if you got fired from your job? None. What difference does it make to them if you gained 20 lbs. back from your last diet? None. That's because our pets love and accept us at the soul level, in a way that's primal and simple—just like the universe itself. So, as silly as it might seem, the next time you're struggling with accepting an issue in your life, ask yourself: *Will this matter to my dog?* If not, then it shouldn't matter to you.

Hidden Agendas

Like self-love, you don't have to DO anything to achieve self-acceptance. It's more about what NOT to do. Just stop resisting everything in your life, and you will, as a by-product, automatically enter a state of self-acceptance. Resistance doesn't have to be outwardly forceful. Most of our resistance is stealthy and hides behind the scenes in our minds. Yes, resistance is bitter self-hatred that many people carry around, but more often than not, we disguise it as "goals" we want to achieve in the future. If we cling to the idea that everything will be wonderful when the ideal weight, perfect partner, great job, or big house enters our lives, we're in a state of resistance concerning our present situation. We have not accepted it. Having goals is a great thing, but when they keep us from living in the present, they prevent us from fully accepting this moment. The best way to discover if your goals are preventing you from complete self-acceptance is to ask yourself: *What if I **don't** achieve* _____? If you have an emotional response to that question, then the issue is creating a hitch in your complete self-acceptance. If you can say, "*Well, it would be great to achieve that, but if it doesn't happen, things are good now. So, that's okay.*" Then, you know you're living from a place of self-acceptance in the present moment.

Detachment to outcomes and freedom from expectations is the key to self-acceptance. It also relieves us of an incredible amount of stress. "Goals" is such a charged word. It implies a fighting or striving for something "better" than what is in the current moment. It automatically implies that what is, is not acceptable. Don't get me wrong: Goals are great and give us reasons to get out of bed in the morning and better our lives. I feel, however, it's better to have *preferences* for our lives instead of angst-ridden goals. Preferences still give us something to work toward, but don't carry the same pressure. We know that even if a situation doesn't work out the way we prefer, everything is still good, because the other option is okay, too.

LET THERE BE

One of the greatest lessons on self-acceptance can be found in the creation parable. We've all heard how the story begins. The declaration was made, "Let there be light." Then, there was. The key word is *let*. It wasn't try, make, work, wish, or construct. Light was *allowed* to exist, and so it was. All creation happens in an environment of true self-acceptance because the new is allowed to come into being. We don't have to DO anything to bring it. We just have to let it come. Let it be. When we let it be, we enter a sacred space of peaceful surrender. It's the quintessential "let go and let God" moment where we know we'll be okay either way, because we're okay right now.

Don't confuse acceptance with approval. The good news is that you don't have to like certain things in your life. You just have to allow them to be. There's a difference. It's like having a bad houseguest. As much as you dislike him, you don't bother with fighting him because you know he's going home in a week anyway. So, you accept his presence and stay out of his way because you know his existence in your life is temporary.

RESPONSE & ABILITY

Self-acceptance means honoring our mistakes. It means understanding that our current situation is in perfect balance in a perfect universe. It's not "wrong" or "bad." It's just a particular place to where a series of choices has led us. We can always make new choices. Self-acceptance means not blaming ourselves or others and owning 100% responsibility of our current situation. Don't confuse surrender and acceptance with quitting or throwing in the towel. Nothing could be further from the truth. When we accept ourselves just as we are, with full responsibility in the present moment, we take our power back. Responsibility gives us the *ability* to *choose* our *response* to something in a *creative* way and bring about change to a situation *as it is now*. The only way to do this is from a present-moment consciousness of self-acceptance. It is the key that unlocks the door of your contraction and will lead you into the next expansion. As poet Robert Frost said, "The best way out is always through."

III. SELF-FORGIVENESS

~~~

"An eye for an eye leaves the whole world blind."
—**Mahatma Gandhi**

"He who is devoid of the power to forgive is devoid of the power to love."
—**Martin Luther King, Jr.**, *civil rights leader*

"He who cannot forgive breaks the bridge over which he himself must pass."
—**George Herbert**, *English poet*

It's not possible to love someone unconditionally if we don't accept them, and it's impossible to completely accept them if we hold *anything* against them. That's why the key to love, the all-powerful creative and healing energy of the universe, is **forgiveness**. If we intend to bring about any positive change in our lives, whether it be losing weight, finding a life partner, or health, it must begin with forgiveness. The power of love is the power that heals. It is the very fabric of the universe. If we intend to use it consciously through our thoughts and beliefs to create the lives we desire, we must access it through the gift of forgiveness.

A Course in Miracles teaches us that all problems in our lives come from some state of non-forgiveness. Quite literally, the healing power of love cannot flow to these areas of our lives because the prerequisite for love *is* forgiveness. It's been said that holding a grudge or harboring hate and resentment for anyone is like drinking poison and waiting for the *other* person to die. Long after the "perpetrator" has moved on, you're still reliving the incident, while he hasn't given it a second thought. The issue no longer bothers him, but you continue to infect your cells with massive amounts of negative energy and messages that create lethal chemical changes in your body. You are, in fact, slowly killing yourself with the poison of unforgiveness.

BLESSINGS IN DISGUISE

I am not assuming that forgiveness is easy. It's not. That's why forgiveness is the ACTIVE portion of the healing process. Acceptance and love are PASSIVE. We arrive at them organically and peacefully *after* having done the real work that lies in forgiveness. Human beings can behave in very inhumane ways toward each other, and I'm not implying that forgiveness will happen overnight. What we understand about the Law of Attraction, however, can help us re-frame the memories that hurt us and see that the problems, and even the perpetrators, were blessings in disguise.

Much of what we dislike about ourselves, including our false, limiting beliefs, is unconscious to us. That doesn't mean, however, that they have to remain invisible to us while they wreak havoc on our lives. Our magnetic, frequency-based universe uses the Law of Attraction to show us, through outward signs those beliefs we're holding inside. Remember, there is no "out there." Every person and situation in your life has been attracted to you by a belief you're holding about yourself. It's the universe's way of saying, *"Hey, you don't think you're worth much! That's bad. So, I'm going to send you a boyfriend who treats you that way. I want you to become aware of that so you can change your mind and get the guy you really deserve!"*

Every person who comes into your life, regardless of whether you deem them a positive or negative influence, *is reflecting some part of you*. It can't be any other way in a magnetic, frequency-based universe. If you enter a room with 200 people, every single one of them reflects a part of you. They must, or by universal law, you couldn't be there.

LIFE COACH

The universe is always trying to raise our attention about our beliefs by sending people into our lives to reflect them back to us. In this light, we can see that these people aren't really a jerk boyfriend, controlling boss, or manipulative sibling. Those are all judgments that keep us mired in self-righteousness and unforgiveness. These people are, in fact, our teachers. Forgiveness comes easier if we can look at them as our life coaches. They're making an appearance in our lives to show us we're harboring negative beliefs that need to be changed so we can live the kind of lives we deserve. They're doing us a great service.

You may scoff and say, *"How is being in an abusive marriage for 20 years a great service?"* With compassion, I would say that the first incident of abuse *was* the universe's message. After that, it was your choice to maintain the old belief that you didn't deserve better and stay. I'm not blaming the victim. In a frequency-driven universe, there are no victims, just personal responsibility and the power to change. We will be hurt by people. That's part of life, but it's akin to the ancient proverb: *Pain is inevitable. Suffering is optional.* We can choose to abandon judgments in these situations and remain aware, looking for the signposts of how to improve ourselves, or we can perpetuate our own suffering by clinging to a blaming, victim consciousness. If we choose the latter, we must realize that as long as we fail to accept the lesson, the "teacher" will remain in our classroom.

Sometimes the message our teachers bring isn't so direct. A cheating spouse may be revealing to you beliefs that you think men are untrustworthy or that you don't really believe in monogamy. He or she may also be revealing something more subtle to you. How are you "cheating" yourself in your life? Are you cheating yourself out of personal time, not pursuing your real dreams, or working for a salary below what you deserve? It's really up to you to examine how someone has hurt you, and where it may apply in your belief system. It's not always as literal as you may realize, but the connection is there.

People who hurt us are often sent to us as a way to release huge amounts of pent-up emotional energy. They're a trigger device. They press all our worst buttons. It's the soul's way of allowing our emotional dam to break before all that anger or pain creates major problems for us, usually health-related. In so many ways, the people that hurt us are our saviors.

STEPS TO FORGIVENESS

There are three main steps to forgiveness: honoring the self, feeling the experience, and re-balancing the event. It's important to go through each step, particularly when it's difficult to see any positive message being provided by the person who has hurt us.

Honor the Self

Take the time to write out the entire incident of what happened. It doesn't matter how long it takes or how many pages you fill up. Don't be diplomatic. Don't be concerned with being fair or analyzing the issue. This is not an intellectual exercise. Let your emotions flow freeform–style, with no fear. No one is going to read this. Simply put your heart on the page as you experienced everything. This is your chance to tell YOUR side of the story.

Feel the Experience

Imagine the person is sitting in front of you. You can use a photograph if it helps. Read "your story" aloud as if the person were hearing you. Feel free to go "off the page" and speak what's in your heart. Let your feelings flow freely. Don't try to manufacture any specific emotion, but do NOT suppress any that arise. The idea is to FEEL this entire experience. Speak, scream, cry, or yell at this person for as long as you need. It's very important not to simply recite the sequence of events, but to tell this person how their actions made you FEEL because of what they did. Be brave. Tap into the feeling and give it a voice!

Don't be afraid to become angry. Anger can be a very healing tool. It gives us access to our underlying pain. Too many times, people who claim to be "enlightened" say that becoming angry is beneath them. I call that dangerously suppressing your emotions. Anger gives us a voice. It allows negative energy to flow THROUGH us and exit instead of lodging inside. It's a contraction that's leading us to the expansion of relief and forgiveness, if we follow its lead and don't bottle it up. There is a myth that there are "good" and "bad" feelings. Those terms are judgments. The only negative feeling is one that is suppressed. Feeling fierce anger for 20 minutes can be extremely healing. Being mired in anger for 20 years because we're afraid of feeling it is completely different.

Don't just recite your story. Get your body into it. Our memories are stored in our bodies, not our brains. If you need to pound the sofa with your fists, do it. If you need to scream, do it. It's important to be vocal, especially for women. For too many generations, women have been suppressed from voicing their opinions and having their say. As a result, many women experience weight gain due to problems with the thyroid gland, which unsurprisingly lies in the vocal energy center of the body, the throat.

Beware of being too easy-going when someone hurts you. Be honest and open with your feelings. You don't have to explode all over someone. Just be forthright with how you feel in the moment. Too often, we pretend that "it wasn't a big deal" or "it wasn't that bad" when someone hurts us. So, we say nothing. We cut the forgiveness process short and dishonor ourselves. We sweep our emotions away too quickly and don't give ourselves a chance to fully process the experience on an energetic level. YOU have to FEEL something before you can FORGIVE something. Otherwise, what is there to forgive at all? As author Mignon McLaughlin said, "What we forgive too freely doesn't stay forgiven."

Re-balancing the Event

Only **after** you've honored yourself and fully discharged the emotion of the situation can you begin to put it into a balanced context, knowing what we know about how the universe works. Stand back from the situation and answer these questions:

1. What belief about myself could this person be revealing to me?

2. Have I been shown this belief from other people in other circumstances?

3. If so, why didn't I react appropriately when I received those messages?

4. This person provided this experience so my life could be changed for the better in what way?

5. What experiences have I had since the incident that verify this improvement?

6. This person has been my teacher in what way?

It's important to remember that any time you become upset, it's about as perfect a lesson regarding your spiritual psychology as you'll ever get. It's like your soul is waving a big red flag, screaming, "THIS IS IT. ATTENTION! THIS IS THE PROBLEM. LOOK HERE!" If we choose to go inward instead of reacting outwardly, we have the chance to heal the place inside us where this pain exists and reclaim our power.

Once you've re-balanced the event, you can see its perfection in a perfect universe. With this information, you can complete the forgiveness release below.

Dear _____,

I understand that you came into my life as my partner in learning a powerful lesson. You helped me discover my false belief that __ _____. Even though _____ had to happen for me to understand this, I am grateful for the gifts it has brought me and how it has bettered my life in ways such as _____ _____. I understand that this was the best way for me to make this change, and that on the soul level, you chose to help me. I am grateful to you for this gift and know without judgment that your actions came from a place of pure love. I forgive you for any temporary pain I experienced and ask forgiveness for any pain I caused you. Thank you for being my partner in this healing experience. I release it and we are both free.

This exercise can be quite profound, and release happens immediately. Other times, it can take a bit longer. Do it as many times and for as many people as you need to. In any case, these kinds of realizations and reframing help us remove our victim stories from our memories. When there are no victims, then there is nothing to forgive any longer. Still, sometimes people will ask, *"How do I know if I've really forgiven someone?"* As humans, we never really forget anything. So this is what I believe: If you can recall the incident, but there is **no** emotional charge to that memory, then forgiveness has taken place.

Like love, the power of forgiveness is not limited by time or space. You don't need to have someone in your life to forgive them. They don't even have to be alive. The energy shift that happens inside of you when you forgive registers across the universal energy field instantaneously and creates a frequency shift in all the parties involved immediately. It *is* that powerful.

Forgiving the Self

As hard as it can be, forgiving others can pale by comparison when it comes to forgiving ourselves. Forgiving others is truly a form of self-forgiveness because, as we forgive those who hurt us, we simultaneously reconcile with those parts of ourselves that we'd become disconnected from.

Even so, we must learn to treat ourselves with the same compassion that we extend to others. The main goal of self-forgiveness is to release guilt and shame. Guilt implies *I did something wrong.* Shame suggests *there is something wrong with me.* Each is a negative belief based on a false perception, a misidentification or missed understanding.

We assume guilt unnecessarily when we take on too much or, quite often, completely undeserved responsibility for something. Guilt is like a punishing parent. It's where all those internal "shoulds" come from. Somehow we *should* have known better, *should* have done something more, *should* have stepped in, or *should* have tried harder. As a result of our "neglect," the outcome of the situation is *our fault.* Nothing could be further from the truth.

If we follow our guilt patterns back far enough, we can see that, like everything else in life, they begin in our childhood. As children, we often think we can make things better. We can make them "right" in our household. When the situation turns out differently than we expected, we take all the unnecessary blame. *If only we'd behaved better, then our parents wouldn't have gotten divorced. If only we'd tried harder, they would have chosen us over the alcohol.* It's these kinds of irrational thoughts that keep us assuming all kinds of responsibility that doesn't belong to us in adulthood. Even when it does, it's blown completely out of proportion. How many times have you said, *"If only I'd been a better mother/father, then my child _____?"* Yes, parents have immense responsibility. When a child is grown, however, he must take responsibility for his own choices.

They key to releasing guilt is to realize that everyone is doing the best they can at any moment with the knowledge they have available to them at the time. That includes you! Look back at yourself at 25 and think about some of the biggest mistakes you made. Would you make those same decisions now? No, because you KNOW better. Give yourself this same allowance today. Realize that there is no way you could make the same mistakes again. You're literally a new person living at a completely different level of consciousness.

Forgiving others is key to forgiving ourselves. As we forgive those who've hurt us, we automatically release the negative beliefs about ourselves that we've attached to the incident. Perhaps you can forgive your husband for leaving you because you now see that his action came to teach you how to be independent for the first time in your life. It gave you freedom! With that realization, you could automatically release the irrational guilt of *"I should have been a better wife and spent more time at home."* Forgiving others is truly a gift we give ourselves in more ways than one.

NEW AGE GUILT

Once we realize the power we have in our thoughts and feelings, we often feel overjoyed with a renewed sense of freedom that we can consciously create our lives. That's usually followed up with what some people call New Age Guilt. It's the feeling of, *"Oh no. That means I brought all the abuse, job loss, bad health, weight gain, and debt on myself. I did it with my negative beliefs. It's all my fault."*

There are no victims in life. If there are no victims, then there can't be any "bad" guys. That means no one is at fault. Everything is happening the way it's intended. With new knowledge come new results. You have the tools now to consciously create what you choose. Everyone is doing the best they can. Through forgiveness, you begin to see how your "problems" have a much higher purpose and actually work to your advantage. With that insight, you might even celebrate your bumps in the road. Remember, guilt "lives" in the past. People who suffer from guilt are always looking backward. The most effective way to dissolve all self-blame connected to guilt is to live with present-moment awareness. In the NOW, there is no past, and guilt has nothing to feed on anymore.

SHAME ON YOU

Shame disguises itself in our lives as the feelings that tell us we're "not enough" of something. Sometimes, we can overcompensate by bragging or lying about ourselves to people. We try to make others feel small in our company. Other times, we constantly do for or give to others in frequent or inappropriate ways because we feel that just our presence isn't enough to keep someone interested. We have to "buy" love. We feel that if we show up exactly as we are, no one will love us, so we have to put on airs. It's the root of all insecurity— the thought, *"There's something wrong with me."*

Shame is the product of abuse and/or neglect. It's the result of our love being rejected, or our trust being violated. The most difficult experiences to forgive are almost always connected to shame because they affect us at the very base level of our self-identification. Forgiving those who have shamed us is certainly possible. People do it all the time. It does require, however, an ability to rebalance the incident from a perspective that some may not be ready to do.

THE GREATER GOOD

Considering the universal principles we've been discussing, someone might easily say, *"I understand how my thoughts and beliefs create my life. I can see how I draw things into my experience based on them. Even so, how can a defenseless child attract a sexual predator into their experience?"*

A great deal of weight gain is the result of such abuse. That's a valid question and there is an answer, although some aren't always ready to hear it. Like attracts like in this universe. That principle is irrefutable. We also know that people are brought into our lives as our teachers, not enemies. It isn't only one person who does the learning in such interactions. Each person in a negative situation is *both* the teacher *and* the student, giving a lesson and receiving one in return. Understanding this, we can see that these negative situations are almost like partnerships designed for our spiritual growth. I believe they are.

A partnership is built on an *agreement*. Two people come together and decide what needs to be done and how to do it. Then, they set about their *plan* to accomplish it. I believe that as eternal souls it is our purpose to expand God consciousness through our individual experiences, both positive and negative. We decide, even before we are born, which lessons we'd like to learn and who would be our best teachers in those areas. We bind with other souls, in contracts of love, to teach each other the lessons we'd most like to learn—even though the process may be temporarily painful for one or both of us.

Perhaps one of the lessons someone wanted to learn was acquiring self-confidence. So, they partnered with another soul who agreed to be born as the controlling mother who they would need to overcome. Maybe another soul's desire was to experience overcoming intense guilt, humiliation, and loss of freedom. So a different soul agreed to be the recipient of his abuse that would ultimately send him to prison. In his work, *Flipside: A Tourist's Guide on How to Navigate the Afterlife*, author Richard Martini explains how these people have actually been our dearest friends for eternity and agreed to incarnate with us over many lifetimes in different roles so we could help each other grow in different ways. Martini says these people belong to the same "soul group." He believes this is why we meet certain people throughout our lives who we feel like we've known before, or carry a strong sense of familiarity for us.

What about newborn babies? They couldn't possibly be creating their circumstances. They can't even speak. Remember that your consciousness/ soul is eternal. It has no beginning and no end. A child's consciousness is completely intact, even in the womb. Just because a newborn cannot speak doesn't mean it's not thinking thoughts. It must. Thinking is a function of consciousness. We make the mistake of assuming infants are somehow less intelligent than adults because they cannot speak. To believe so would be putting God and consciousness into a very small box, indeed. On the contrary, their consciousness is as complete as yours or mine before they even enter the world.

It's not important nor is it necessary to understand what spiritual contract you may have made with someone who has hurt you. All that's necessary to start the forgiveness process is to be *open to the idea* that there is, in fact, a much greater good at play in what seems to be a very dark situation.

NO FREE PASS

This does NOT mean that we are to condone harmful behavior. Everyone is responsible for their own actions. When we put negative experiences into this light, however, we can begin to see that our "chaotic" world has never been out of balance at all, nor can it ever be. With our myopic human senses, we tend to classify everything as either "good" or "bad." In reality, it's impossible to have both.

If the universe is ONE, how can a unified whole be divided against itself? How can it be two things when it is ONE? It can't. All there is is love, and everything comes from love. Even our most painful experiences are born out of love. If everything is happening for a greater good, as I believe it is, then nothing "bad" really happens.

Off the Hook

Now that we understand that our negative experiences—and those who participate in them—are actually happening for a greater good (our spiritual evolution), we can let ourselves off the hook. We can forgive ourselves for things like marrying the wrong guy, losing a job, not accomplishing the goals we had in our younger years, and anything else. We can give ourselves a break and see that, within the scope of a larger, divine plan, we walked away from these experiences with some very valuable gifts for a better life. We can be kind to ourselves and realize that anyone else in those positions would have acted in the same way that we did at the time, with the amount of understanding and knowledge that we had. We fulfilled our role as the student, and now we get to move on. In addition to the above forgiveness exercise for others, below is a simple statement you can use for yourself. It's a simple dialogue you can have to establish trust between you and your higher self again.

> *(Your Name), please know that I understand why you _____. Given the circumstances at the time, anyone with the amount of knowledge you had would have made the same choices. You did the best you could. You're a different person because of that experience and would certainly make different choices today. The fact that we made it through that experience is a testament to your strength. I love you and thank you for that. I recognize that this experience was for our growth and that we did nothing wrong. We can now move forward without judgment, guilt, or feeling like a victim because we fulfilled our part in the divine plan perfectly. It is done and we are free.*

Higher Ground

It's only by examining the painful experiences of our lives from a higher perspective that we can begin to make sense of seemingly senseless acts. We can begin to release ourselves from the negative emotion that binds us. In fact, it can be reassuring through this understanding that not a single second of anyone's suffering has been in vain. It's only from space, looking down on Earth, that we finally see the shape of our world isn't even close to what we once thought it was. It's all about perspective.

REALITY CHECK ... THE PILLARS OF PERSONAL CHANGE

✓ Love is the most powerful force in the universe; the highest frequency we can experience.

✓ The bioelectrical field of the heart is 5,000 times stronger than that of the brain.

✓ Love doesn't exist in a vacuum. In an attraction-based universe, we must *give* love to receive it in return. It's our relationships that heal us.

✓ Loving others is Self-Love because we are all ONE and that love returns to you!

✓ The void in our hearts is only filled when we put love in. Don't worry so much about getting all the dark emotions "out." Darkness disappears when light enters.

✓ God is love. Nothing imperfect can exist in the presence of God, so healing is the application of love to the places within us that are hurting.

✓ To love someone or something, you must accept it unconditionally.

✓ Self-Acceptance is allowing everything to be okay as it is right now.

✓ You don't have to *approve* of something to allow it to be.

✓ Having preferences for our lives instead of angst-ridden goals helps us remain in a place of Self-Acceptance in each moment.

✓ All creation and healing happen in an environment of Self-Acceptance because the new is *allowed* to come into being.

✓ True Self-Acceptance is letting go and letting God.

✓ We cannot accept anyone or anything if we hold a grudge against them and, therefore, cannot love them. We access the healing power of love through forgiveness.

✓ Forgiveness is ACTIVE and leads to the PASSIVE states of acceptance and love.

✓ Our "perpetrators" are our life coaches. They make us aware of negative beliefs so we can change them!

✓ Seeing someone as our teacher removes judgment and helps us forgive more easily.

CHAPTER 14

MY STORY

When I started this book, I hesitated about sharing my story. I wasn't sure if I could be that vulnerable with so many of those who know me, and even those who don't. I realized, however, that I've been called to be a healer in this life. It brings me a sense of purpose and great joy. Sometimes, the most powerful piece of information we can give anyone is our own example. If my story can provide guidance for your own healing journey, then I offer it freely with equal parts love and gratitude. I also believe that when you're facing the biggest challenge of your life, no piece of advice is nearly as helpful as the story of someone who has "been there."

MIDNIGHT MESSAGE

I was in my second year of medical school and had gone to bed early after another grueling day of lectures. My mind was ready to explode from the overload of information we'd received that day on the renal system, which includes the kidneys and urogenital organs. I was exhausted and just wanted to forget about it all until the next morning. I was asleep almost as fast as my books hit the floor.

It was 2:00 a.m. when my eyes shot open. From a dead sleep, I'd been thrust into total alertness. Virtually at the same time, I heard a very clear voice in my left ear. *"Check yourself."* I didn't even question it. Instinctively, I somehow knew what to do. I got up, went into the bathroom and performed a testicular exam. There it was. A lump on my left testicle. I froze. I thought, *"Where did THIS come from?"*

BACK TO BEFORE

I was born in Iran, a land that is as beautiful as it can be culturally restrictive, and at times, politically unstable. In an unpredictable environment such as the one I was growing up in, my protection against the dangers outside my home should have come from the love I was receiving inside it. It didn't. My earliest memories include being physically and sexually abused in the most deplorable ways by people I loved and trusted. As a result, I grew up with an enormous sense of guilt and shame from the punishments I was receiving. Because I grew up with a fundamentalist idea of a punitive God, I was certain I deserved the abuse. There *must* be something wrong with me; otherwise, people wouldn't be treating me this way.

In order to survive, I did what we all do. I stuffed everything down inside. I turned off my ability to feel and pretended it wasn't happening, just so I could get up and face another day. I couldn't fight back. I never had my say. I certainly couldn't talk to anyone about it, least of all a God, who as far as I was concerned had sanctioned the punishments against me. I felt completely alone.

OF MIND AND MEN

Because of the guilt and shame I was carrying, I walked into my adolescence with a complete lack of self-empowerment. I couldn't protect myself or those I loved from the ongoing violence in my home. As a result, I soon found it very difficult to assert myself in any area of my life. I couldn't conduct myself in any way that was direct, powerful, assured, or confident, especially with girls. The aftermath of the sexual abuse left me questioning my sexuality. Even though I knew my inherent orientation was heterosexual, my young mind couldn't reconcile how such a thing could happen to me and what it meant, if anything, about my sexual identity. Ultimately, these mental debates left me struggling more with my sense of masculinity than my sexuality. How could I be a "real man" if I couldn't protect myself or my loved ones? I was weak and ineffectual. It wasn't possible for me to be a real man and allow such sexual abuse to happen. I was submissive and a coward. It was these ideas that colored every area of my life, from participating in sports and making friendships to dating. I had no role model in my life to show me what a real man was. I had the images from TV and movies, and judging from those, I definitely wasn't one.

CULTURE SHOCK

Seeking better opportunities, my family decided to move to the United States. On the surface, that might seem like a good thing. Many years later, it would prove to be. In the beginning, however, it was a culture shock of epic proportions laid on the shoulders of a boy whose back was already about to break.

I knew we came to America for a better life, but I didn't know what "better" meant. All I knew was what was familiar to me. To be a 12-year-old Iranian boy dropped in the center of an American high school with absolutely NO frame of reference for the culture or language is beyond terrifying. It's traumatic. For a child who so desperately needed protection, I found myself once again in a frighteningly vulnerable position. I couldn't communicate with anyone about any of my needs, not to mention looking completely different from every person in the school. In my child's mind, it was like being on another planet, and in reality, I might as well have been.

THE BEST INTENTIONS

By the time I reached high school, I had absolutely no friends. I had no connection with anyone outside my home. There was no support structure anywhere for me. I desperately wanted to connect with someone, anyone. Just to have a semblance of a conversation, even with my broken English at that point, would have made me feel like I belonged somewhere. I would have had a sense of value in someone else's eyes.

At that time, I was doing a lot of weightlifting in the gym. I noticed all the football players would come in and workout between practices. In high school, everyone knows the football stars are epitome of masculinity, and they always get the prettiest girls. Everybody wants to be friends with the IN crowd, and you can't get more popular than a football quarterback.

So, I made a plan. I got an old yearbook and looked up each player. I cut out their pictures and used them like flashcards to memorize their faces and practice saying their names. I thought that once I could call them by name fluently, it would be the spark to start a conversation and the introduction to what could be lasting friendships. I kept the pictures in my wallet so I could test myself during study halls and other downtime.

In the meantime, I approached Coach Kaiser, head of the football team, to ask him where I could get a pair of proper lifting gloves because I'd begun to develop calluses on my hands. He suggested that I speak to Robby Blake, the captain of the football team. To my teenage self, Robby Blake was a rock star. He was super-human. He had a body like a Greek statue and he knew it. He regularly showed off by walking around campus in nothing but a Speedo bathing suit, almost always with at least two girls on each arm competing for his attention.

One day, I mustered my courage to approach Robby during his usual campus tour with his posse of admirers. I expressed myself well enough to convey that the coach referred me to him about getting some gloves and he was very glad to help. He said that I should follow him to his locker and he'd find a pair for me. After he found my size, he said the gloves would cost $10. *This couldn't have been easier. What was I so afraid of?* Robby seemed to be such a nice, regular guy.

As I opened my wallet to get the money, all the football players' pictures that I'd cutout from the yearbook tumbled onto the floor. Robby looked at the pictures. He looked at me. Then, he took a step back and said, "Oh my God. You're a faggot!" From that moment on, my life went from bad to a level of worse I couldn't even have imagined. My limited English wouldn't allow me to defend myself properly or explain. It wouldn't have mattered. After that, the entire school believed I was gay. I have many gay friends and patients today, but in high school during the time I attended, people were NOT nearly as educated or accepting about the realities of sexual orientation. I even hesitated to print Robbie's actual quote because of the slur he used, but it's important to understand the intensity of the scarlet letter I would wear for the next several years, at least in the minds of the other students.

BAD TO WORSE

Students made a sport out of taunting me. Girls would come into the gym in very revealing clothing and pretend to drop a quarter on the floor in front of me. In what seemed like slow motion, they would bend over to pick the coin up and in the process, rub their backsides into me in a very provocative way. As a gentleman who also came from a very religious family, I always opted to step aside and not behave in an inappropriate manner. That's not what everyone else saw. They just continued to point at me say, "See. I told you he's really queer."

The kids were relentless in calling me all sorts of things I didn't understand. It was only after I spoke with Coach Kaiser that I found out the terms were all colloquialisms for being homosexual or gay sex. With no one to turn to and no way to process this whole experience, I reacted in the only way I knew how. I stuffed it all down and tried to maintain as low a profile as I could to make it through the next three years. When I think about all the gay teens who are ostracized so mercilessly in high school and ultimately commit suicide, my heart aches for them. I know what they're going through because it happened to me, and I wasn't even gay. I would urge young people today to share their pain with anyone who will listen. I didn't have anyone and, quite honestly, I don't know how I survived it. I've always believed, though, that what you reveal, you heal.

Too Much Information

For the next four hours, I sat at the computer in my college apartment scouring the internet for every possible thing that could have been wrong with me. I scared myself to death with far too much information. Perhaps the scariest thing was that I had no medical insurance.

I called my brother, who was a physician in San Diego at the time. Knowing how medical students are notorious hypochondriacs, he wondered if I was imaging things. I assured him I was not. I'd delayed pursuing my education while I supported him during his time in medical school at the University of Southern California. He was now returning that favor and was able to get me some insurance coverage. I immediately made an appointment to be examined.

Opting Out

It was cancer. After "that word" was spoken, I didn't hear anything else the doctor was saying. His lips were moving, but it was like everything was happening underwater. This was happening in 1997, the same time Olympic gold medalist figure skater Scott Hamilton had gone public about his battle with testicular cancer. He'd endured extensive surgery during his experience. Not long afterward, Tour de France champion Lance Armstrong made his announcement about his testicular cancer, and how it had spread to his lungs and brain. There seemed to be no hope. I was panic-stricken.

After seeing a team of urologists and oncologists, the plan included removing all the lymph nodes in my gut in addition to extensive rounds of radiation and chemotherapy. I thought to myself, *"Here I am in the most medically-advanced country in the world, and this is the best modern medicine has to offer me? This is it?"* I saw very quickly that from a strictly medical point of view, the choice they were offering was that I had no other choices.

Seeing there was no real choice in the outer world, I chose to go within for my answers. I intuitively felt that the same guiding intelligence that brought the cancer to my attention in the middle of the night could tell me how to heal from it, as well. I decided that I *did* have another choice. I opted out of all the conventional interventions and decided to go "off the grid" of commonly accepted therapies. I decided to trust my life with a power that seemed to know more about this process than I did; but in the hands of who or what I was placing my trust—I had no idea. That's when everything changed.

Something More

Taking a leap of faith off a cliff with your life in your hands is not easy, especially when friends and family members are claiming you have a death wish. Trying to calm my anxiety over my condition, while debating terrified family members, only compounded my stress and sense of isolation. In standard fashion, all the doctors wanted to do was give me anti-anxiety medication and schedule my surgery. Intuitively, I knew pills and surgery couldn't give me the answers I was seeking. They couldn't give meaning to what was happening to me.

In the midst of fighting my fear and family members, I was visited by the same ghosts from my past. *This is God punishing me. I deserved this.* Here I was again, re-evaluating what it was to be a man. Was I a man just because I had two testicles? Was I a man simply because I could father a child? What made a "real man," and was that the kind I wanted to be?

When it comes right down to it, there are only two kinds of people on Earth. Before nationalities, political parties, religions, and race, we are either a man or a woman. That's all. When the very last objects we use to identify ourselves are stripped away, what's left? When something cuts this close to your personal identity, it forces you to re-examine the fact that you are something beyond even that. I was beginning to believe I was.

TAKING OFF

I had to do something about school. I couldn't do what I felt I needed to do and deal with the stress of medical school at the same time. The dean was cordial, but very matter-of-fact in telling me to take a month off, have the surgery, and come back. I knew what I needed, but couldn't assert myself with him. Driving home, I regretted my lack of courage. I thought, *"Is this the most humane way to treat myself, or anyone in this position? Is this what I really want?"* After I got home, I called the dean and told him I was taking a year off.

In such a disempowering situation, I chose to take my power back. I immediately shaved my head and all body hair as a symbol of the decision-making authority I still had over my life. I wasn't going to lose it to chemotherapy. I did it myself mostly as a symbol of letting everything go and jumping off into the unknown.

I started off backpacking through Mexico, and soon found myself studying ancient healing traditions with a Curandero, shamanic healer in the mountains. This experience led me to Guadalajara and Veracruz, Cordoba, where I read everything I could get my hands on about healing and natural medicine. I was astonished at all the healing modalities I or even my professors back at school had never heard of. I was introduced to anthroposophical medicine and herbal interventions of all kinds. I became a voracious student, and couldn't process all the information I was receiving fast enough.

Ultimately, my journey led me to Himachal Pradesh in Northern India, where I learned Vipassana meditation. I studied with Dr. Doshi, the personal physician of the Dalai Lama, and discovered Tibetan medicine. I was amazed not just by the herbals they were providing to people, but also the *way* they were being prepared was just as important as the element itself. Meticulous attention was given to when the herbs were harvested, how they were laid out to dry, as well as lunar and solar cycles. It was a way of administering medicine that was completely unknown to me. It became very clear to me that the real solution to any ailment didn't come in a purple pill.

This knowledge took me back to a re-emergence in yoga, massage, and osteopathy. Even though I was a student of osteopathy at the time, it was this *direct experience* that was showing me how the elements of mind, body, and spirit were equally integrated to facilitate healing. What did it **really** mean to foster healing from a higher perspective? This wasn't just the BIG picture I was seeing. This picture had no frame, no limits, no judgments, and no assumptions about any one modality being more credible than the other. The miracle was in how they were working together.

Although I couldn't see it at the time, this experience was to shape how I would practice medicine for the rest of my career. I firmly believe I had to have this direct experience. I had to have been in the position of the patients I would eventually be treating to be able to create interventions that would work organically *with* their bodies' natural healing process and nurture their spirits. I will tell you, there is NO teacher like direct experience.

MAKING THE CONNECTION

Back home, I immersed myself in German New Medicine. I started to understand how traumas affect us on a biological level, and how certain experiences remain in our cellular memory. In this fascinating modality, experts give patients CAT scans without contrast and can tell them what their primary and secondary emotional conflicts are with regard to their health.

That's when I made the connection between my emotional and physical health. I began to realize how much trauma I had really gone through. I knew it was bad, but after I reached adulthood, I figured I'd survived and could move on. Once I took stock of it all, I saw how I numbed myself to get through those times. It wasn't that anything got better. I just stopped allowing myself to FEEL in order to survive, but I was starting to see that feelings buried alive always come back to haunt you.

It became clear to me that all the suppressed emotions from my life traumas were finally surfacing. Since the majority of that pain was sexual in nature—from my sexual abuse and struggle with masculinity to my sexual humiliation in high school—it was no coincidence that the spot my pain chose to manifest was in the male sexual center: the testicles.

COMMON SENSE & SURRENDER

While I was making these connections, I still had trouble reconciling my idea of God, deservingness, and how I brought all this on myself. That all changed when I confided in my dear friend, Gary. Upon hearing what I'd been through the last year, he invited me to dinner. That night, he shared his personal story and it brought me to tears. It taught that no matter how perfect it looks on the surface, everyone in the world has at least one story that can break your heart. He said, "I don't know about you, but the God I have chosen is not a punitive God. It is a loving God. It's the only thing that makes any sense. He who hasn't loved hasn't known God." That simple but powerful statement quenched my fear in an instant, and remains an inspiration to me to this day.

After that conversation, I released something that left me with a deep sense of surrender. No matter how this journey ended for me, I **knew** there would be love, peace, and grace during the entire process. No matter what they might have to cut out of my body, I could never be less than a man . . . or less than whole.

BREAKING THROUGH

Days later, after my daily meditation, I picked up a pen and just started writing in a stream-of-consciousness way. I had no agenda or idea what I was to write. I simply picked up the pen and let my spirit tell me what was on my mind. To my astonishment, a torrent of memories started pouring out onto the paper. Some I could recall and others I was completely unaware of up to that point. After each meditation session, the floodgates of my heart would open even wider. As I transferred my pain to the page, I could literally feel its corresponding ache in my body. I could feel the tension in my jaw or the ache in my back. I could finally feel where all the negative energy had been hiding in my physiology for so many years as it was released. No one needs to tell me your biography becomes your biology. I knew in that moment that it was completely real.

As I released my pain, I knew instinctively the next step had to be forgiveness, or the negative energy would return to these places in my body. I had to go back and forgive all those who had hurt me and stolen my innocence along with what should have been the most precious times of my life. It was because of them I felt shameful, guilty, and unworthy, but now I had the capacity to forgive. I'd finally made room for it in my heart where the anger and pain had once been.

I didn't feel like I had to locate all the people from my past. Somehow, I knew that if I spoke to them from my heart, out loud, that they could hear me on the level of the soul. If we're all truly connected and all is ONE, then they *must* be able to hear me. I know they did. As I spoke honestly of my feelings about what they did to me and offered forgiveness for their actions, I could feel the energetic release happen. It was almost like a cord being cut that connected me to them and the experience. The memories that were most highly-charged for me took more than one conversation, but it eventually did happen. It was real and I was finally free.

GOING HOME AGAIN

There was one person I did decide to find. It was Coach Kaiser. Because my abuse in high school had been so relentless for so long, I felt that a return to that place now as an adult man who was not afraid or ashamed would provide me with a level of healing that would allow my inner child to put that experience into its proper perspective. I could finally ask the coach why he didn't speak up for me to the other kids when I couldn't speak for myself. Why hadn't he intervened in a way that could have prevented much of the abuse I'd received? I could also tell him how much I admired him as a role model in other ways. It was a fascinating conversation that I'm convinced was healing for both of us.

As I moved through the forgiveness process, the strangest thing happened. I regained a sense of control over my life. I had developed a deep sense of trust in myself and in the spiritual intelligence that guides me even though I'd been diagnosed with cancer. At a time when I should have been at the heights of anxiety, I was experiencing the deepest peace I'd ever known. I knew these hurtful experiences came into my life for very specific reasons, and as I was discovering the Soul lessons, they were falling away. I was reminded of Victor Frankel, the brilliant doctor who survived the Nazi concentration camps of WWII. He attributed his very survival to changing his perspective on what was happening to him. He said that it's the meaning we give to what happens to us that determines everything else. We must find the courage to go "off the grid" of our limited understanding of "good" or "bad" and open ourselves up to the possibility of healing based on a much greater plan. In my office, I have a poem by the Persian poet Rumi that says, "Out beyond wrongdoing and rightdoing, there is a field; I will meet you there." That is where "off the grid" exists. That is the place where there is no judgment, no duality, only wholeness and THAT is where healing lies—in the place of pure love.

That was my life between 1997 and 1998. Today, I am cancer-free with no surgery, radiation, or chemotherapy. I am a physician, and I knew the realities of my condition back then. I also knew there was a much greater power that exists beneath all true healing if I could just access it. I know now that, because I trusted myself, I was really trusting the power that made me, and that divine guidance led me to real love. That's why I never think of myself as having had cancer. I always say I had *canswer* because it was the key to healing my heart and ultimately my body. It was my roadmap back to my innocence, honor, and masculinity. I finally understand what it really means to be a man. Now, I can teach that to my son.

CHAPTER 15

YOUR LARGER DESTINY

~~

"Everyone thinks of changing the world, but no one thinks of changing himself."

—**Leo Tolstoy**, *author*

"Every action in our lives touches on some chord that will vibrate in eternity."

—**Edwin Hubbel Chapin**, *minister*

"To put the world right in order, we must first put the nation in order; to put the nation in order, we must first put the family in order; to put the family in order, we must first cultivate our personal life; we must first set our hearts right."

—**Confucius**, *philosopher*

Take a moment and try to think of yourself as not existing. I didn't say to imagine not being alive. That's different. Try to imagine yourself as never existing . . . ever again. You can't. Why? It's because, inherently, you already know you are an eternal spiritual being. You are that singular energy that makes up everything in the universe, vibrating at a specific frequency that makes you . . . you. Since energy can never be created or destroyed, it means that you have always been and will always BE.

Knowing the only thing that moves this energy into form is mind, there **must** have been an initial thought or desire that brought *you* into your current form, the life you're living right now. Because we know the universal laws are governed by our free will to use them, that means the choice to bring you into this life to live this specific experience was made by and could ONLY have been made by . . . you. You chose to be here.

MOVIE IN MY MIND

You might say, *"I chose to be here? Why would I choose to be overweight, sick, or poor? If I made the choice, why don't I remember making it?"*

I believe life is a classroom and we are all here to learn specific lessons of our own choosing. It can be no other way if free will reigns supreme in a universe based on love, as I believe it does. That means you and I made choices at the spirit level as to which lessons we'd like to learn most in this lifetime. We also chose the best stage on which these lessons would play out, along with the perfect supporting actors to fill out the experience. We don't remember our divine nature or even making this choice because *we didn't want to.* We chose to have the veil come down between us and the divine to give the illusion of separateness. We knew the only way to really learn how to swim was to be thrown into the deep end. We're so terrified we're going to drown that we've taken our eyes off the lifeguard who's ready to jump in the pool at a moment's notice. We don't see the loving protection that's never left us for a single moment because we've been paddling too hard most of the time. How do you prefer to see a great movie? In the dark! Why? It's because it makes it feel more real . . . like you're actually there. We chose to live our lives in "the darkness" of forgetting our spiritual essence because it would make watching the film a richer experience.

SAME LESSON, DIFFERENT PATHS

This isn't to suggest that your life is predetermined and you're stuck being over overweight or sick. You're not. Your consciousness and free will remain the only determining factors of how your life unfolds. Many of us choose to learn the same lesson but in different ways. One soul that has chosen to learn humility might become a missionary in Africa, while another opts to be a famous politician who experiences a scandalous fall from grace. We may not be able to change our current circumstances directly, but we can choose new circumstances indirectly by choosing how we react and feel about our current situation. This is how real change is created. Some of us may be learning the same lesson in more difficult ways than others, but the length of time it takes us to learn that lesson by raising our own consciousness and passing through it is entirely up to us. You did NOT come here to suffer in order to learn. Why not take the lesson pain is trying to teach, and start learning from joy instead?

MISSION POSSIBLE

You had an even bigger reason for choosing this life besides spiritual growth. The nature of the universe is eternal expansion, and it's fueled by continuous growth: yours, mine, and every other human being's. Remember, we're all connected. There is only ONE source from which we all emanate. This source is experiencing this growth through you, *as* you. It's like one of those huge mirror balls that hang above a dance floor. There's only one ball, but when it's illuminated it reflects hundreds of tiny lights that dance around the room as it rotates. You and I are each one of those reflected lights dancing across the universe of time and space.

Our individual spiritual growth not only expands our own consciousness, but it expands the collective consciousness of the entire human race, as well. It's the microcosm affecting the macrocosm again. As you heal, you actually heal the world. You are like a single cell in the "body" consciousness of the human race. Every time a cell heals, the body gets better. Your mission isn't just to heal your own life, but to heal the world as you do it. So much for being insignificant! Your healing is absolutely essential for world healing. That's the bigger reason you chose to be here, at a time when our world is in dire need of healing more than ever before. You wanted that big of a challenge because you KNEW you could do it. Because your success means imminent healing for the world, the universe is on pins and needles waiting for you to succeed. You may not see it, but there are legions of souls in eternal grandstands somewhere cheering you on. The universe *wants* you to succeed. It's depending on it so much that it's given you all the tools to virtually guarantee it. That's more than a mission possible. It's a mission accomplished!

BACK FOR MORE

Nobody gets the short end of the straw. Nobody gets the eternal leftovers after all the "good stuff" has been handed out. You meticulously designed your life and chose the challenges you're facing right now because you knew they would bring you the greatest reward . . . and you knew you could do it. We tend to become anxious and focus on the surface conditions of our problems because we believe life is temporary. If we don't straighten everything out in this run, well then it's all over. We've lost our chance to do, be, and have all the things we wanted. We become nearsighted by staring at the ticking clock we all attach to our lives, believing that time is real and it's running out fast. We panic and take life far too seriously because we think we're missing our one shot.

The truth is upon our death, we simply return to the ONE again. We haven't gone anywhere. We've just made a frequency change that's less dense than the one that corresponds to the world we're currently living in. That's all. We're eternal. Nobody does everything in one lifetime. The kinds of experiences a spirit can have are infinite. Growth depends on direct experience, and since growth is our spiritual specialty in helping the universe expand, common sense would dictate that we do not live just one lifetime. The "clock" isn't real and the mirror ball will continue to rotate above the cosmic dance floor for infinity. That's why as difficult as your situation might be right now, you might think you'll be better off never coming back. I wouldn't bet on that. Life in all its manifestations is such a delicious experience that, next time around, you might want to appear as another point of light but on the other side of the ballroom.

Because life is a divine dance with many turns on the dance floor, you can be at peace knowing there really is a higher plan guiding the entire process. Have confidence and know that all is well. Whether you know it or not, you're exactly where you need to be, and your progress is perfectly on schedule.

FINDING FAITH

In difficult times, faith is essential to creating change. Like love, faith is completely misunderstood. Most of us have seen televangelists bantering on screen, "I believe! I believe! I believe!" It's almost as if they're trying to convince themselves that what they believe is actually true instead of simply stating it to their congregation. Faith is not boastful, strident, or insistent. Faith is simple. **It's understanding**. When you understand something, then you KNOW it to be true. It needs no campaigning because its validity simply is. We only fear what we don't understand.

It's unfortunate that most of us are taught that great faith—the kind of faith that changes lives—is a special talent of mystical sages, saints, and clergymen. This is ridiculous. We all have great faith. The problem is that we allow fear to take over, and fear is faith . . . just in the wrong things.

Now that we understand how the universe works and that we're holding ALL the cards, we don't have to fear circumstances anymore because we know we create them. We can also re-create them at will, based on how we direct our thoughts and attention. Faith is quiet confidence. It's knowing that, even though we may not see our desire manifested yet, the unseen energy of the universe is at work, following our lead, reorganizing itself to bring it about. It's the spring flower ready to break through the thawing winter earth.

CONSISTENCY IS KEY

Just keep going. Don't stop. Set your intention for the life you choose and don't look back. So many times, we give up because we haven't seen what WE would call progress. We end the journey too soon, when our destination was right around the corner. The truth is you won't know how you're going to get to your destination until AFTER you've arrived there. If a friend gave you driving directions to a place you've never been before, when would you know those directions were correct? You certainly couldn't rely on your physical senses, looking for landmarks and such. The route would be completely foreign to you. You wouldn't know the path was the right one until AFTER you reached your destination. Don't worry so much about "how" you're going to get there. Universal laws are designed to handle the details. Let them do it! Your job is to clean your emotional house and then aim your thoughts, feelings, and attention in the direction of your intention.

Don't step on the scale every day. A watched pot never boils. You're also telling the universe that you don't really have faith in its process. You need to check up on it. You're not sure it's working. The universe is listening, and it's going to make sure it's not working for you because that's what you're expecting. Stay focused on your intention, do your work, and you will get there. It was once just a trickle of water that would carve away the stone that would become the Grand Canyon.

GET A MOVE ON

Faith is knowing that this process isn't a secret. It's a science. It works all the time, every time. As long as you're thinking, you're using it. You've just been using it in the wrong direction. Sometimes, we don't move at all because we don't know which direction to take. Just move. Now. Your single choice will create momentum in the universe that will begin to guide you. It's like the GPS navigation system in your car. It's very powerful and will get you to your destination with perfect accuracy every time . . . but you have to put the car in gear and MOVE it first for the system to work the way you need it to. If you happen to take a wrong turn, your spiritual GPS will tell you which way to turn to get back on course. Faith is trusting the process because you understand how it works.

We easily have faith in so many things but don't realize it. When you order a pizza for delivery, you know that it usually arrives in 30-40 minutes. You make the call and let it go because you know how the routine works. You don't get on the phone every ten minutes, calling the pizza shop saying, *"Is he coming? Are you sure he's coming? How far away is he? Will he be here in the next five minutes?"* You place your request. You expect and plan for its arrival and leave the details of how it gets to you to other powers. That's faith. Order the pizza and begin setting your table for its arrival.

FAITH VS. HOPE

Many times people believe they're using their faith in the right way when what they're actually doing is hoping. To hope is to want the best but plan for the worst. Hope is uncertainty about how things might turn out. Hope believes there are greater forces against you, but that there's a chance you *might* win out. Hope is wishing. Faith is knowing. The universe is listening.

LIKE MINDS

Be sure to surround yourself with people who believe in you. This will help you keep the faith through setbacks and be valuable partners in your progress. Politely dismiss the well-intentioned, fear-based urgings of family and friends. Set your goal as high as you like. The universe's abundance is endless and will pay any price. How much are you asking? Forget about being "realistic." Actor Will Smith said, "Being realistic is the fastest road to mediocrity." Sir Edmund Hillary didn't set a "realistic" plan to only scale Mt. Everest halfway up because that's as far as any human being had ever climbed. He intended to go all the way to the top . . . and he did!

THE POWER OF GRATITUDE

Be sure to give thanks all along the way, for your small victories and even when you feel you've hit a plateau. Gratitude is a very powerful frequency and draws to you more things to be grateful for. When you really take stock of all the things you have to be grateful for, your perspective changes immediately and you see just how rich your life really is. If you start with the things you take for granted, like being able to see, hear, and walk, you'll recognize how abundant your life already is. Meister Eckhart, the German philosopher, has said, "If the only prayer you ever say is 'Thank you,' that will be enough."

CHAPTER 16

A FINAL WORD

~~~

Healing is a singular destination with many different routes. You and I may be going to Phoenix, but we'll be taking completely different roads to get there if you're in Denver and I'm in Los Angeles. I could gather ten patients together, each dealing with the exact same condition, and yet, each one will have a completely different reason for experiencing it that's unique to them. I've shared some very valuable tools with you, including my own journey to healing, but only you can provide yourself with the specific directions you need to get there. Trust the higher intelligence that guides you. It will lead you there, if you allow it.

I recently performed a lengthy phone consultation with a very successful businessman. He found himself dealing with cancer he thought he'd rid himself of through surgery years ago. Now, it was back. For two hours, I explained to him the concepts I've shared with you. His continued response was, *"Yes, but what's your success rate?"* Like any good businessman, he was only thinking in numbers, basing everything on logic alone. He wanted a formula, a one-size-fits-all approach, something he could just DO and get over with.

I explained to him that healing is like the most powerful supercomputer ever created. It holds all the answers to every question you could ever ask. If you don't educate yourself on how to use the computer, it's useless to you. It will just sit there and do nothing unless you understand how to operate it. When you do, the success rate really is 100%.

During my healing journey, I was hiking out in the middle of the desert in Joshua Tree National Park, and it began to rain. At first, I was upset because

I was miles from my car and would be soaked by the time I got back. All I could do was surrender to that moment. Once I did, my perspective on the rain completely changed. I began to revel in its strong scent and cool sensation. I let it fill me up and wash me clean. It was then that the rain gave me an acronym for how simple healing really is. We must **R**ealize the problem, **A**ccept it, and then **I**nvestigate what it's trying to tell us about ourselves. Lastly, we must ask ourselves what it is we **N**eed to make that part of our soul complete again. On the surface, the answer will appear to be different for all of us but underneath, it will always be based in love because love is the only thing that heals. It's the only thing that ever has.

We have more information about health now than we've ever had in history, and yet, people are sicker than they've ever been. Information **never** healed anyone. If that was the case, all those warnings on the back of cigarette packs would have stopped millions of people from smoking. That never happens. It's because information doesn't heal people. *Inspiration* does. Use the information in this book to become inspired and connect with your spirit. When you go within and seek what your heart is hungry for, you will find it . . . and you will be fed.

As you and I continue our life journeys, we help each other heal because we are ONE. My healing lifts you up and yours does the same for me in return. We really *are* in this together. No one is alone. It can't happen any other way in a universe that is already complete. Everything is ONE thing. That thing is love and you'll find it . . . within.

THE PROGRAM

~~~

THE EXERCISES

Each exercise in this program is designed to either get you into a **forgiving place** or a **feeling place**. The forgiveness exercises will focus on forgiving others as well as yourself. They may bring up a lot emotion for you. That's okay. In fact, it's good. Do your best to stay open to whatever comes. Don't try to generate any kind of expected response. Healing can happen in a quiet way as easily as it can in a dramatic one. Let whatever comes forward be honest and real. Give yourself the permission to allow it and know you are safe in the process. If you feel you need to focus the forgiveness exercises on more people than what's asked of you in the program, feel free to repeat them at the end. In fact, feel free to repeat any exercise that you find particularly beneficial once the program is finished. You may also repeat the program in its entirety at any time.

The feeling exercises are designed to get your body into the act, to start re-programming your cellular memory and subconscious by participating in experiences that help you feel the way you want to feel in your new body. Don't worry if they feel awkward, especially in the beginning. Your mind is like a cup of coffee that you've only stirred in one direction. When you begin to stir it in the opposite direction, there is a brief moment of chaos in the cup. The ripples are choppy and don't know which way to go. Eventually, the liquid gets going just as easily in the other direction. Be prepared for this brief moment of discomfort, but don't be discouraged by it!

THE CORE

In addition to the featured exercise, each day includes a core set of activities that contain the principles we've discussed in this book. They are a crucial part of the program and must be done every day as described. They include:

- **Morning Meditation**: Sit quietly in a comfortable chair and focus on your breath. Don't engage any thoughts that arise. Just let them pass through your mind and come back to the breath. Keep your eyes closed and have a watch nearby. This helps you check the time without having to open your eyes all the way to look for a clock. If you find sitting in silence difficult at first, you may repeat a short mantra. Upon inhalation, think but do *not* say the word "so." During exhalation, think the word "hum." So Hum is a healing mantra that means "I am that." 15 minutes

- **Movement / Exercise**: Any type of movement that is enjoyable and involves your whole body. Walking in the park, dancing, etc. 30 minutes

- **Affirmation**: Choose an affirmation that works for you. Don't try to convince yourself that you're thin right now. Your mind will reject that statement. Just be sure it is in the present tense and you feel no resistance when you speak it. You might choose, "My healing is in process and my body is following freely." Repeat silently or aloud as needed throughout the day.

- **Visualization**: You can do this any time. Right before bed is ideal. Close your eyes and imagine yourself in your ideal body doing all the things you'd love to do. Be sure to put yourself actively in the scene with a first-person point of view. This shouldn't be like you're watching yourself do all these things. You're actually doing them so you can feel all the sensations, sounds, tastes, noises, and sights to their highest degree. Revel in this. It must be fun! At the end of your chosen scene, imagine yourself on a stage. Family and friends approach you, each giving you a flower and saying, "Congratulations." Psychologists have found this word provides a very strong sense of completion. 5 minutes.

- **Gratitude**: Write down five things that you are grateful for that happened today. Can be done any time.

- **Evening Meditation**: Same as morning. 15 minutes

Nutritional Components

Each day comes with one nutritional recommendation. There are no calories to count, foods to weigh, or menus to follow. Incorporate each recommendation into your normal eating schedule for *that* particular day. If you find the change resonates with you, then carry it over to the next day in addition to the new recommendation. If not, simply move onto the next day's suggestion. The recommendations are designed to add healthy changes incrementally, and to introduce you to foods in interesting ways that are new to you.

Supporting Your Digestion

I said this book isn't about food and it's not. I think you've gotten that message by now. Even so, I wanted to provide a very basic, but powerful recipe that will help support your digestion and increase your metabolism throughout the next 40 days.

Rejuvelac is a lacto-fermented tonic that was popularized by nutritionist and author Ann Wigmore during her recovery from cancer. It's a simple drink made from nothing but wheat berries and water that's full of lactobacillus bacteria, minerals and enzymes, which are essential for a speedy metabolism and thorough digestion. When we digest our food fully, we are completely nourished by it and experience less hunger cravings. Unfortunately, most of the food we eat today has no probiotics, very little nutrition, and no enzymes, so we end up staying in a chronic state of craving because, although we're over-fed, we're actually under-nourished. Do your best to add a few daily servings to whatever meal plan you decide is best for you. If you can do this, you'll not only experience a shift in your digestion, but also your moods since healthy intestinal flora is essential to how we feel.

Rejuvelac Recipe

- **3 cups organic rye berries**
  *We're using rye here to limit gluten, but organic wheat berries work just as well.

- **1 large glass jar with clasping glass lid and rubber seal**

- **Purified, spring or distilled water**
  Do not use tap water. The chlorine, fluoride and additives will not support the fermentation process.

- **A strainer**

1. Pour the rye berries into a strainer and rinse them thoroughly with purified water.

2. Place the berries in the jar and cover them with water until the water surface is 2-3 inches above the berry line. Wrap a towel around the jar to keep the light out. Do

not seal the lid. Leave it open, but place a paper towel over the top so the berries can breathe. Let sit for 12 hours.

3. Pour the berries into the strainer. Rinse them again. Place them back in the jar with more purified water. Wrap the jar in the towel and put the paper towel back on top. Let sit for another 12 hours.

4. Pour the berries into the strainer once more. Rinse again. This time, put the berries back in the jar with NO water. Wrap the jar in the towel. Put the paper towel back on top. Wait 24 hours.

5. By now, you should see tiny white sprouts breaking through the ends of the rye berries. Over the next 24 hours, leave the berries in the dry jar, but be sure to rinse them twice!

6. When the sprouts are ½ inch in length, fill the jar with purified water again to about 4 inches above the sprout line.

7. Seal the jar by clasping the lid closed. Do not wrap it in the towel this time. Let sit for 2-3 days. During this time, carbon dioxide will build up in the jar. This is good! That means your probiotic cultures are alive! Just swirl the jar a couple of times per day without opening it to dissipate some of this excess gas.

8. After three days, strain the Rejuvelac into clean glass jars or bottles.

9. To make another batch, simply pour water over the sprouts once again and wait three more days. After this second harvest, the berries are spent. Throw them away and start again at step one.

Some Things to Remember:

- The Rejuvelac should be a slightly cloudy, golden color.
- It should taste pleasantly tart without being too sour.
- It will be lightly effervescent and bubbly, almost like a carbonated soft drink.
- It should not smell "off" or like rotten eggs. If so, the batch has failed, most likely due to contamination in the jar or impurities in the water.
- The fermentation works best when done in a room that remains relatively cool, at around 75 degrees.
- For the best results, have 8-oz before breakfast, after lunch, and after dinner.

A COMMITMENT TO MYSELF

I understand that I am complete, a divine soul, God consciousness here on Earth to realize my perfection through a life of abundance and joy. I know my key to manifesting this abundance lies in my ability to use my God-given creative power with complete awareness and total accountability. I accept full responsibility for my life as I commit to this program for the next 40 days. My new life begins today. I promise you, _____, that I will honor this commitment to you with courage, persistence and faith. I celebrate with you the amazing life we have already begun to create not just because we can but because we deserve it!

Signature _____

Date _____

DAY 1

THE CORE

Morning Meditation: 15 min.

Exercise/Movement: 30 min.

Gratitude List: 5 things

Evening Meditation: 15 min.

Visualization: 5 min.

CELEBRATE!

You read that right! All you have to do today is celebrate any way you like. That includes whatever you'd like to eat. No restrictions. Just feel the joy of change that is already reorganizing energy in unseen ways to manifest itself in your life.

DAY 2

THE CORE

Morning Meditation: 15 min.

Exercise/Movement: 30 min.

Gratitude List: 5 things

Evening Meditation: 15 min.

Visualization: 5 min.

YOUR SIDE

Honor the Self

On a sheet of paper, write out the entire incident of what happened between you and the person you feel has hurt you the most in life. It doesn't matter how long it takes or how many pages you fill up. Don't be diplomatic. Don't be concerned with being fair or analyzing the issue. Simply put your heart on the page as you experienced everything. This is your chance to tell **YOUR** side of the story.

Feel the Experience

When you are finished, imagine the person is sitting in front of you. You can use a photograph if it helps. Read "your story" aloud as if the person where hearing you. Feel free to go "off the page" and speak what's in your heart. Let your feelings flow freely. Don't try to manufacture any specific emotion but do NOT suppress any that arise. The idea is to FEEL this entire experience. Speak, scream, cry, or yell at this person for as long as you need. It's very important not to simply recite the sequence of events, but to tell this person how their actions made you FEEL because of what they did. Don't be afraid to become angry. Anger can be a very healing tool. It gives us access to our underlying pain. Be open to whatever comes up.

Don't just recite your story. Get your body into it. Our memories are stored in our bodies, not our brains. If you need to pound the sofa with your fists, do it. If you need to scream, do it. It's important to be vocal, especially for women.

When you are finished, destroy the letter in a way that has finality. Don't just throw it away. Burn it, shred it or some other way that is empowering to you.

That's all you need to do. Take as much time as you need to settle yourself. It's important to reset yourself emotionally by doing something you love, like calling a friend or taking a short walk.

NUTRITIONAL RECOMMENDATION

Subconsciously, our food tastes better and satisfies us more if it's presented in an attractive way. Advertisers know this! Take time with your food and make it beautiful. No eating leftovers out of the pot today! Eat *at least one meal* on your best china plate garnished with parsley or a slice of citrus. Drizzle some melted butter over fish and sprinkle it with hand-cut fresh herbs. Lay some green onions across your soup and dust the rim of the bowl with dried herbs as if it were served in a restaurant. Look at pictures in recipe books for ideas and have fun. These are simple changes that will not only make your food look better, but taste better and satisfy you more.

DAY 3

THE CORE

Morning Meditation: 15 min.

Exercise/Movement: 30 min.

Gratitude List: 5 things

Evening Meditation: 15 min.

Visualization: 5 min.

PLAYING THE PART

Choose a person you admire, who has the type of body, personality, and life you want for yourself. This person lives the kind of life you see yourself living at your ideal weight. It could be an actor/actress, politician, humanitarian, or someone you know personally.

Your subconscious won't buy the fact that you're somebody else because it already knows you're you! A great way to sidestep this limitation is to imagine you're wearing a virtual, lifelike mask of this person's face. You're still you, but you get to pretend and play behind the safety of your celebrity mask, giving you a sense of freedom and protection. This also takes the pressure off of you feeling like you have to do an impersonation of someone.

For the rest of the day, in all your interactions with people, behave and respond as your chosen role model would. Get your whole body into this. FEEL how they walk. HEAR the inflection in their voice when you speak. Laugh like they do, and carry their confidence. Even the most subtle changes in behavior during this exercise can be very powerful.

NUTRITIONAL RECOMMENDATION

Color is food's way of signaling to us that it has health and healing properties. The brighter the color, the more antioxidants and other beneficial properties the food carries. For every meal today, be sure you can count at least five different colors on your plate. Avoid meals that are all "beige" with just meat, bread, pasta, potatoes, gravy, etc.

DAY 4

THE CORE

Morning Meditation: 15 min.

Exercise/Movement: 30 min.

Gratitude List: 5 things

Evening Meditation: 15 min.

Visualization: 5 min.

REBALANCE & RELEASE

Re-balancing the Event

After you've honored yourself and fully discharged the emotion of the Your Side exercise on Day 2, you can begin to put it into a balanced context. Stand back from the situation and write out the answers to these questions:

1. What belief about myself could this person be revealing to me?

2. Have I been shown this belief from other people in other circumstances?

3. If so, why didn't I react appropriately when I received those messages?

4. This person provided this experience so my life could be changed for the better in what way?

5. What experiences have I had since the incident that verify this improvement?

6. In what way has this person been my teacher?

Once you've re-balanced the event, you can see its perfection in a perfect universe. With this information, complete the forgiveness release below.

Dear _____,

I understand that you came into my life as my partner in learning a powerful lesson. You helped me discover my false belief that _____. Even though

_____ *had to happen for me to
understand this, I am grateful for the gifts it has brought me and
how it has bettered my life in ways such as* _____
_____. *I understand that this was
the best way for me to make this change and that, on the soul level,
you chose to help me. I am grateful to you for this gift and know
without judgment that your actions came from a place of pure love. I
forgive you for any temporary pain I experienced and ask forgiveness
for any pain I caused you. Thank you for being my partner in this
healing experience. I release it now and we are both free.*

The universe loves symbolic gestures and this last step is designed to elevate your feeling of release. Get a helium-filled balloon of your choice. You can find them at most dollar stores, party supply stores, or florist shops. Go to a quiet, private place that is special to you. It could simply be your patio, apartment balcony, backyard, or a park. Read your release statement to this person out loud with reverence, respect, and gratitude. When finished, release the balloon. Open your arms as wide as they will go. This gives a strong sense of expansion. Watch the balloon drift away and feel your burden become lighter as it gets higher and higher and eventually disappears.

NUTRITIONAL RECOMMENDATION

Our taste buds get trained by eating the same foods and flavors all the time. They come to expect them and can create unhealthy cravings. It's time to wake up all your taste buds. In each meal today, incorporate savory spices you've never tried before. If you can find fresh, organic herbs, the depth of flavor and experience will be much more satisfying. Look for ways to incorporate things like sage, thyme, rosemary, star anise, cardamom, caraway seeds, or even curry into your dishes. If you have an ethnic restaurant near you that serves Indian, Persian, or Thai food, be bold and give it a try. You'll be surprised how your cravings for sweetness will diminish if you're stimulating your palate with deep, savory flavor.

DAY 5

THE CORE

Morning Meditation: 15 min.

Exercise/Movement: 30 min.

Gratitude List: 5 things

Evening Meditation: 15 min.

Visualization: 5 min.

THE ROYAL TREATMENT

Take time today and treat your body in a special way. Run a hot bath. Be sure to use some good bath salts or essential oils in the water. Light candles and allow yourself to luxuriate in the sensory-rich experience you've created. You can even play relaxing music. Don't hurry through this. Take the time to explore your body in the bath. See how the water trickles off your curves. Explore your body as if you were seeing it for the first time.

When you're done, apply body lotion or a powder that you particularly like. Do this slowly and nurture yourself as you move your hands across your body. Make this a sensual experience. Communicate to your body that you love it through the quality of your touch. The healing quality of touch is quite powerful. Too often, we treat our bodies badly, look at them with disappointment, or just take them for granted. Tell your body how much you love it through your sense of touch. Think of all the wonderful things it does for you to keep you healthy, all the functions you never seem to notice and be grateful.

Afterward, put on something that makes you feel beautiful. It could be a nightgown, lingerie or just a robe. Relax and do something enjoyable, like reading a book or watching your favorite TV show.

Nutritional Recommendation

Eliminating distractions means we can be fully present with our food. For today, do *nothing else* while eating. That means no watching TV, driving, reading, or talking on the phone. Sitting in a chair, simply eating a meal at a table will bring new awareness to your relationship with food. See what comes up for you. Your body will thank you, too, as all that secondary energy you normally expend will be redirected to helping with digestion.

DAY 6

THE CORE

Morning Meditation: 15 min.

Exercise/Movement: 30 min.

Gratitude List: 5 things

Evening Meditation: 15 min.

Visualization: 5 min.

ME & I

Set two chairs facing each other and be seated in one. Look across from you and imagine your 8-year-old self sitting in the other chair. This person is beautiful and innocent. Sit quietly until you can clearly visualize him or her there. Some people call this an "inner child" exercise, because in many ways the person you are visualizing in the chair is you at your core: pure, loving, trusting—much like a child.

When you're ready, greet your other self and ask a simple question. It might be, "Hi there. How are you today?" Keep it very simple. Once you've asked the question, switch chairs. Feel the inner part of you that is childlike, honest, and open. Take your time. Find the feeling and then answer the question from this emotional place. Do not censor yourself and try not to stop to think about what your answer will be. This works best when you answer freely and let your words flow with your stream of consciousness.

You may be surprised at what comes out. You many answer, "Fine. Do I HAVE to do this?" or, "Terrible. I wanted pizza all week for lunch and you made me have a salad." Whatever the response, just let it come. When the impulse to respond stops, switch chairs and assume your adult perspective again. Respond to the remarks, but never admonish the child or try to negate their feelings by explaining anything. You might simply say, "We don't have to do this right now. Is there anything else you wanted to do or say?" or, "I know salad isn't very tasty but maybe we can find something better tomorrow that we both like. What would you suggest?"

Keep the dialogue going. It's designed to reveal thoughts and desires you didn't know you had and reconnect with the innocent part of yourself that you've disassociated from. When we treat ourselves badly through unhealthy behaviors or even negative words, we alienate our inner child and intuition. After a while, the child no longer trusts us because we've ignored him/her for so long, and eventually doesn't show up when we need it the most. This exercise helps reconnect the adult logical side of ourselves with the child creative side, and integrate our sense of self.

NUTRITIONAL RECOMMENDATION

Fruit is healthy and provides many antioxidants and fiber. It can backfire on you if you're choosing fruits that are too sweet. Sugar, much more so than fat is the real weight loss enemy. Your body treats sugar the same way whether it's from a doughnut or a banana. Have a serving of sub-sweet fruit with every meal today such as lemons, limes, grapefruits, sour grapes or green apples. You'll get the benefits of fruit without all the sugar.

DAY 7

THE CORE

Morning Meditation: 15 min.

Exercise/Movement: 30 min.

Gratitude List: 5 things

Evening Meditation: 15 min.

Visualization: 5 min.

A PHONE CALL AWAY

Pretend you are in your ideal body. Pick a department store, salon or any retailer that provides a good or service that you'd love to have but your weight has prevented you from purchasing. You're going to call this location and have a conversation AS IF you were already in your perfect body.

You might want to call a department store and speak with a clerk in the dress department. Ask them if they carry a specific designer that you like. Tell them that you're looking for a size 8, 10, or whatever your ideal is. That's YOUR size and you really love their style. Can they suggest any other designers that might look good on you, because you have a traditional hourglass figure? Keep the conversation going. The idea is to FEEL yourself speaking these words and to put them out into the universe where they begin to move and change things. Have fun with this. Daydream out loud. You might even call a few other retailers, too.

If you're a man, you might want to call a gym and ask about memberships or contact a company that sells bodybuilding supplements. Ask a bodybuilder what he recommends for building more muscle and creating muscular definition. You could even call a personal trainer inquiring about his rates and workout advice.

Play this part as much as possible. You're not lying. You're role playing. You're giving your mind and body a new blueprint of how to think and act as a thin person. Remember to have fun. It has to FEEL good!

Nutritional Recommendation

More calories usually means more ingredients and additives. For each meal today, do not eat anything that contains more than five ingredients and especially anything you can't pronounce! The simpler food is, the fewer calories it contains, and the healthier and easier it is to digest. As a general rule, the fewer calories a food item has, the more nutrient-dense it will be, and vice versa.

DAY 8

THE CORE

Morning Meditation: 15 min.

Exercise/Movement: 30 min.

Gratitude List: 5 things

Evening Meditation: 15 min.

Visualization: 5 min.

YOUR SIDE #2

Honor the Self

On a sheet of paper, write out the entire incident of what happened between you and **the second person** you feel has hurt you the most. Be blunt and honest. This is your chance to tell **YOUR** side of the story.

Feel the Experience

When you are finished, imagine the person is sitting in front of you. Read "your story" aloud as if the person where hearing you. Feel free to go "off the page" and speak what's in your heart. Let your feelings flow freely. Don't try to manufacture any specific emotion, but do NOT suppress any that arise. The idea is to FEEL this entire experience. Get your body into it and scream, cry, or punch a pillow if you need to.

When you are finished, destroy the letter in a way that has finality. Don't just throw it away. Burn it, shred it, or some other way that is empowering to you.

That's all you need to do. Take as much time as you need to settle yourself. It's important to reset yourself emotionally by doing something you love like calling a friend or taking a short walk.

NUTRITIONAL RECOMMENDATION

We all know we're supposed to eat more fruits and vegetables but how much more? The best ratio is 80/20. That means your meals should consist of 80% fruits and vegetables with 20% protein and fat. An easy way to know if your ratio is right is to imagine your plate as the face of a clock. The wedge between 12:00 and 2:00 should be filled with your meats and fats. The rest of the dial should be filled with green and all the other colors of fruits and vegetables. Work this ratio into each meal today. If your "beige" food items extend beyond the 2:00 mark, it's time to reconfigure the arrangement.

DAY 9

THE CORE

Morning Meditation: 15 min.

Exercise/Movement: 30 min.

Gratitude List: 5 things

Evening Meditation: 15 min.

Visualization: 5 min.

HOW ARE YOU?

Ask as many people as you can today, "How are you?" Nearly everyone will reply in some fashion of, "I'm well, and how are you?" When they ask you how you are, that's your chance to put more positive intention out into the universe. You can reply, "I'm terrific. I just lost 35 pounds, and my boyfriend proposed last week!" or, "Just wonderful. I recently booked a cruise to the Caribbean, and I'm so excited to go!"

The idea is to ask people who don't know you personally. Cashiers at the grocery store, postal clerks, or receptionists are a few good examples. Respond with items and activities that you don't think you can do until you lose the weight. You're creating a mental map in your mind that it's already happened when you speak the words. Words are very powerful, especially with the feeling we attach to them. So, be excited about sharing how wonderful you feel because of all the positive new developments you're intending in your life.

NUTRITIONAL RECOMMENDATION

Fermented foods provide us with powerful probiotics and enzymes to aid in digestion. These beneficial microbes actually pre-digest the food for us by breaking it down and making the nutrients much easier to absorb. They also provide excellent byproducts, such as Vitamin B12. Eat a fermented food with every meal today, especially if it contains meat. Good choices include yogurt, kefir, kim chi, sauerkraut, or cultured butter and buttermilk. Beware of most grocery store yogurts and kefirs. Most have cane sugar added after the fermentation process to sweeten them up. Look for one with the least amount of sugar possible. A quality fermented food is not sweet at all, but slightly tangy.

DAY 10

THE CORE

Morning Meditation: 15 min.

Exercise/Movement: 30 min.

Gratitude List: 5 things

Evening Meditation: 15 min.

Visualization: 5 min.

REBALANCE & RELEASE

Re-balancing the Event

After you've honored yourself and fully discharged the emotion of the **Your Side #2** exercise, you can begin to put it into a balanced context. Stand back from the situation and write out the answers to these questions:

1. What belief about myself could this person be revealing to me?

2. Have I been shown this belief from other people in other circumstances?

3. If so, why didn't I react appropriately when I received those messages?

4. This person provided this experience so my life could be changed for the better in what way?

5. What experiences have I had since the incident that verify this improvement?

6. In what way has this person been my teacher?

Once you've re-balanced the event, you can see its perfection in a perfect universe. With this information, complete the forgiveness release below.

Dear _____,

I understand that you came into my life as my partner in learning a powerful lesson. You helped me discover my false belief that _____. Even though

_____ *had to happen for me to understand this, I am grateful for the gifts it has brought me and how it has bettered my life in ways such as _____ _____. I understand that this was the best way for me to make this change and that, on the soul level, you chose to help me. I am grateful to you for this gift and know without judgment that your actions came from a place of pure love. I forgive you for any temporary pain I experienced and ask forgiveness for any pain I caused you. Thank you for being my partner in this healing experience. I release it now and we are both free.*

The universe loves symbolic gestures, and this last step is designed to elevate your feeling of release. Get a helium-filled balloon of your choice. You can find them at most dollar stores, party supply stores or florist shops. Go to a quiet, private place that is special to you. It could simply be your patio, apartment balcony, backyard, or a park. Read your release statement to this person out loud with reverence, respect and gratitude. When finished, release the balloon. Open your arms as wide as they will go. This gives a strong sense of expansion. Watch the balloon drift away and feel your burden become lighter as it gets higher and higher and eventually disappears.

NUTRITIONAL RECOMMENDATION

The three biggest crops in the U.S.—wheat, corn and soybeans—are known as genetically modified organisms (GMO). This means the seeds have had their genes altered in a laboratory so they produce fluffier bread or can survive aerial-sprayed pesticides and assaults from insects. The problem is that once their genes are altered from their natural counterparts, our bodies don't recognize them as food. It might look like wheat, but on a genetic level, our bodies don't see it or treat it that way. This is why so many people have problems with wheat gluten and other grain-based products. It will be a challenge, but for each meal today avoid all corn, wheat, and soy based foods. Read labels and you'll be surprised how many processed foods contain these three ingredients.

DAY 11

THE CORE

Morning Meditation: 15 min.

Exercise/Movement: 30 min.

Gratitude List: 5 things

Evening Meditation: 15 min.

Visualization: 5 min.

DO IT ANYWAY

List three things you don't feel you can do until you've lost the weight. Perhaps it could be go dancing in a nightclub, walk through the door of your local gym to inquire about a membership, take a dip in a swimming pool, or rollerblade. It should be something you've wanted to do but feel it's "only for skinny people."

Pick one of them and do it anyway. Yes, I said do it anyway. I might be frightening at first, but the only way to eradicate fear is to do the very thing that frightens us. When we see we've survived afterward (as we ALWAYS do), we eliminate an old false belief and create a new KNOWN in our mind. Most importantly, you'll be doing the very thing that you've trained yourself to believe that only skinny people can do. Once you begin to do it, your subconscious will begin to reprogram itself to believe you really are skinny because you're doing the very thing only skinny people can do . . . therefore, you must be, too!

NUTRITIONAL RECOMMENDATION

Eating smaller, more frequent meals is one of the best ways to stave off hunger and keep your body's metabolism moving throughout the day. People who eat several smaller meals experience less hunger and maintain a faster metabolism. It also keeps your blood sugar levels stable, making you less apt to overeat dinner because you skipped breakfast and had a meager lunch. For today, eat 5-6 smaller meals instead of three large ones. It might be easier to scale back on your three meals and just add three "snacks" between them. These really shouldn't be full meals, but more like some cheese and grapes or vegetables with a healthy dip.

DAY 12

THE CORE

Morning Meditation: 15 min.

Exercise/Movement: 30 min.

Gratitude List: 5 things

Evening Meditation: 15 min.

Visualization: 5 min.

ME & I

Check in with your inner child again as you did in Day 6. See how he or she is handling this whole process. Remember to keep the questions simple. Don't judge or admonish your innocent self for replying in any particular way. Your goal is to discover how he or she feels, uncover hidden beliefs, and re-establish trust. Remember to not censor yourself and be as free as you possibly can in the exercise. Be sure to ask forgiveness and apologize for anything which your inner child holds a grudge against you, because you're holding it against yourself!

NUTRITIONAL RECOMMENDATION

Most people don't know that they're drinking over half their daily calories! For today, eliminate all processed drinks including soda, coffee, and tea. Create flavorful drinks that cater to your other tastes. If you have a juicer, combining cucumber, celery, parsley, and fennel with some ginger root or mint in 10-oz of water makes a fantastic, light, and refreshing substitute for high calorie drinks. If you live near a health food store, coconut water kefir or kombucha are wonderful fermented drinks that are low-calorie but have a natural bubbly effervescence similar to the carbonation of soda. You can also use juice from the grocery store, but be mindful of the sugar content and *always* dilute it with water. Stick with 100% cranberry or some other non-sweet fruit or vegetable product.

DAY 13

THE CORE

Morning Meditation: 15 min.

Exercise/Movement: 30 min.

Gratitude List: 5 things

Evening Meditation: 15 min.

Visualization: 5 min.

DEAR DIARY

In a journal, make an entry about what happened in your life on a particular day in the near future. Like any diary entry, be sure to put a date on it, but one that's not too far in the future. You might pick a date six months from now.

Imagine and write in as much detail as you can the events that happened on that day in your life at your "ideal weight." You might say that you went to buy something new to wear for a friend's birthday party that evening and everything looked amazing on you. Describe the outfits you put on and how they complemented your body. Maybe on the way out of the mall you grabbed a bite of your favorite ice cream, feeling no guilt whatsoever, and then ran into an old high school acquaintance who commented on how great you look. Later that night, you meet a very interesting person at the party who asks you out on a date for next week.

Think big with this. Have FUN. Feel the excitement of all the day's events as you write them out. Through this exercise, you're forecasting your life, designing it by your intention and the positive energy you're putting out. The more you FEEL this exercise the more you're telling your subconscious that it is how you really are and eventually . . . you will be!

NUTRITIONAL RECOMMENDATION

Losing weight isn't about eliminating fat. It's about avoiding the wrong kind of fat and as much sugar as possible. Humans have been on Earth and eating for over 200,000 years, but Americans have only been consuming polyunsaturated fats—processed vegetable oils—for about the last 100 years.

We all know what's happened with obesity and weight-related illnesses in that time period, as well. Coincidence? I don't think so. These highly-processed corn, soybean, canola oils and margarine are foreign to our bodies. They cause us to gain huge amounts of weight and wreak havoc on our digestive systems that don't know how to identify them as food or break them down. Avoid these fats and any foods that contain them. Choose good saturated fats as they come from nature, such as butter from grass-fed cows, cold-pressed olive oil, and coconut oil in their raw forms or for low-temperature cooking. For high-temperature food preparation, I suggest beef tallow or good old-fashioned lard. Yes, I said it: lard.

DAY 14

THE CORE

Morning Meditation: 15 min.

Exercise/Movement: 30 min.

Gratitude List: 5 things

Evening Meditation: 15 min.

Visualization: 5 min.

COMFORTING TOUCH

When we don't like our bodies, we hide them or speak badly about them because we're embarrassed of them. How would any other conscious being treat you if they knew you were embarrassed of and spoke badly about them? Your body's cells have consciousness, too, and they know how you feel about them! Is it any wonder our bodies don't seem to want to cooperate with us when we want to lose weight? Would you want to help someone who thought so ill of you?

Take some time and lie in bed. Create a relaxing environment by dimming the lights or putting on some soft music. Close your eyes. Start at the top of your head and touch your hair. Let your hands rest there. Feel its texture and thickness. Talk to it. Tell it that you love it and why you appreciate it. Perhaps you love its color, or its one of your best features. Slowly move downward and carry on the same conversation with your ears, eyes, lips, skin, shoulders, stomach, and so on. Don't rush through this. Touch your own body the way a comforting parent would touch a child. Be sincere and realize how much your body gives you that you forget to be grateful for. Appreciate and honor it with love and respect.

In the 1970s, there was a craze of people talking to their house plants. Everyone thought they were kooky because they swore their plants grew taller and greener because of it. Today, we know exactly why that's true! This exercise helps establish a new, cooperative, and loving relationship between you and your body. Love is healing. Give love to your body and it will listen to you!

NUTRITIONAL RECOMMENDATION

Our bodies are designed to perform certain functions in daylight and others at night. Your body literally rebuilds itself during sleep, especially if you're ill. It can't carry on these processes if it's busy digesting food (a daytime activity). For today, be sure to finish eating at 8:00 p.m. That includes flavored drinks!

DAY 15

THE CORE

Morning Meditation: 15 min.

Exercise/Movement: 30 min.

Gratitude List: 5 things

Evening Meditation: 15 min.

Visualization: 5 min.

YOUR SIDE #3

Honor the Self

On a sheet of paper, write out the entire incident of what happened between you and **the third person** you feel has hurt you the most. Be blunt and honest. This is your chance to tell **YOUR** side of the story.

Feel the Experience

When you are finished, imagine the person is sitting in front of you. Read "your story" aloud as if the person where hearing you. Feel free to go "off the page" and speak what's in your heart. Let your feelings flow freely. Don't try to manufacture any specific emotion, but do NOT suppress any that arise. The idea is to FEEL this entire experience. Get your body into it and scream, cry, or punch a pillow if you need to.

When you are finished, destroy the letter in a way that has finality. Don't just throw it away. Burn it, shred it, or some other way that is empowering to you.

That's all you need to do. Take as much time as you need to settle yourself. It's important to reset yourself emotionally by doing something you love like calling a friend or taking a short walk.

NUTRITIONAL RECOMMENDATION

At breakfast we're actually "breaking a fast" from not eating through the night. It's never a good idea to force a heavy meal on your stomach right after waking. Today, drink a 10-oz glass of water with the juice of half a lemon 20 minutes before breakfast. Lemon juice is very alkalizing, cleansing, and will help prepare your digestive system for the coming meal. It also helps to "turn your liver on" for detoxification.

DAY 16

THE CORE

Morning Meditation: 15 min.

Exercise/Movement: 30 min.

Gratitude List: 5 things

Evening Meditation: 15 min.

Visualization: 5 min.

THE BENEFACTORS

In order to manifest anything in our lives, our intention cannot benefit just us. It must benefit others, as well. When we align our intention with making the lives of others better as well as our own, our desire manifests much faster. In the space below, write all the ways you can think of that your weight loss will benefit others. Perhaps your newfound energy will allow you to spend more time with friends, adding enjoyment to their lives. Maybe you'll be able to act as an inspiration to others in their struggle to lose weight. When we give to others, we keep the flow of good things coming back to us. How will your weight loss give to others?

_____

_____

_____

_____

_____

_____

_____

_____

_____

_____

Nutritional Recommendation

Avoiding processed and GMO grains like wheat, white rice, corn, and soy is easier if you can substitute them with healthy alternatives. Quinoa is becoming very mainstream and can be found in most grocery stores now. It's high-protein with all the essential amino acids. It's not a starch like rice, but can be prepared much the same way. Buckwheat is another great choice. It's not a grain, but actually a seed. Amaranth, another high-protein grain, can be found in health food stores. Incorporate one of these into your meals today. It also helps if you soak them in a bowl of water overnight. They'll cook faster and digest better!

DAY 17

The Core

Morning Meditation: 15 min.

Exercise/Movement: 30 min.

Gratitude List: 5 things

Evening Meditation: 15 min.

Visualization: 5 min.

Rebalance & Release

Re-balancing the Event

After you've honored yourself and fully discharged the emotion of the **Your Side #3** exercise, you can begin to put it into a balanced context. Stand back from the situation and write out the answers to these questions:

1. What belief about myself could this person be revealing to me?

2. Have I been shown this belief from other people in other circumstances?

3. If so, why didn't I react appropriately when I received those messages?

4. This person provided this experience so my life could be changed for the better in what way?

5. What experiences have I had since the incident that verify this improvement?

6. In what way has this person been my teacher?

Once you've re-balanced the event, you can see its perfection in a perfect universe. With this information, complete the forgiveness release below.

Dear _____,

I understand that you came into my life as my partner in learning a powerful lesson. You helped me discover my false belief that _____. Even though

_____ *had to happen for me to understand this, I am grateful for the gifts it has brought me and how it has bettered my life in ways such as _____ _____. I understand that this was the best way for me to make this change and that, on the soul level, you chose to help me. I am grateful to you for this gift and know without judgment that your actions came from a place of pure love. I forgive you for any temporary pain I experienced and ask forgiveness for any pain I caused you. Thank you for being my partner in this healing experience. I release it now and we are both free.*

Read the statement out loud and perform the balloon release in a setting that is special to you. Remember to open your arms wide when you release it and watch until it fades out of sight.

NUTRITIONAL RECOMMENDATION

Eating consciously means really getting in touch with our food. Make eating a tactile experience today. Eat only items that you can physically touch: a sandwich, vegetable sticks, etc. Examine how your reaction to food changes when you're constantly coming into physical contact with it.

DAY 18

The Core

Morning Meditation: 15 min.

Exercise/Movement: 30 min.

Gratitude List: 5 things

Evening Meditation: 15 min.

Visualization: 5 min.

Random Acts of Kindness

We're always getting too wrapped up in our problems. We seem to think we're the only one on the planet. One of the best ways to forget your problems and to feel great at the same time is to help someone else. Remember how great it felt to help someone who was completely surprised at your gesture? That's what we're going for today: feeling great through giving. The key in this exercise is to be a secret giver so that the recipient doesn't know where their good came from. It's more fun that way, and the point of this exercise isn't about recognition or taking credit. It's about feeling good through putting good out into the world and making someone else's life better. As a result, your life will be better, too, in ways you won't be able to anticipate.

You might want to pick out a single person at the restaurant where you'll be having lunch or dinner. Approach the hostess and pay for their meal without their knowledge. They'll get a wonderful surprise when they ask for their check. Send someone flowers unexpectedly with no note or even drop quarters in the parking meters of strangers that are about to run out. Every gesture, no matter how small, creates more joy for you and the recipient . . . and even the world.

Nutritional Recommendation

If you choose to have dessert, eat it first before the rest of your meal. Yes, you CAN have your dessert first. Sugar from all foods, including fruit, metabolizes quickly. Other foods, such as meat and cruciferous vegetables, take longer to digest. Eating sweet foods after a meal prevents them from moving through your digestive system quickly, as they get stuck in line behind the heavier foods. This can cause the sugar to stagnate in the digestive tract, creating fermentation and a perfect food source for negative bacteria like *Candida albicans* to flourish. The result is gas, bloating, and irritable bowel. If your meal includes sweet foods, eat them first!

DAY 19

THE CORE

Morning Meditation: 15 min.

Exercise/Movement: 30 min.

Gratitude List: 5 things

Evening Meditation: 15 min.

Visualization: 5 min.

SOW & REAP

The universe is clear. You reap whatever you sow in life. One of the best ways to get what we desire is to give it to others. Remember, everything comes back to you. So, the best way to get what we want is to give it to others or help them achieve it.

Weight takes a toll on our self-image. We don't feel attractive when we're not at our desired weight. We want to feel beautiful. Go through today and shower as many people with compliments as you can. Don't be insincere. You can truly find something about everyone that you can appreciate. You might compliment someone on how beautiful their hair is or how well their outfit goes with their eyes. Tell someone else that she looks great in her dress or that his hat suits him perfectly. When we find the beauty in others, we find the beauty in ourselves.

NUTRITIONAL RECOMMENDATION

Sugar in all its forms will undermine the best weight loss efforts. We can be sabotaged by the hidden sugar in many normally "healthy" foods that aren't perceived as sweet-tasting. These foods are the starches. Although a potato may not taste sweet, it is filled with starch, which is converted into sugar very, very quickly in the bloodstream after consumption. For today, have a "white out" and eliminate all starches from your diet. The easiest way to do this is to avoid any food that is white. This includes white breads, bread products made with enriched flour, white rice, potatoes, and pasta. Blood-sugar levels and calories can be reduced more by this dietary change than almost any other. Preparing some of the alternate grains we discussed will make this change much easier.

DAY 20

THE CORE

Morning Meditation: 15 min.

Exercise/Movement: 30 min.

Gratitude List: 5 things

Evening Meditation: 15 min.

Visualization: 5 min.

TAKING STOCK

Forgiving others is important to our healing, but so is seeking forgiveness from those we have wronged. Unresolved conflicts with others we have hurt can leave us with underlying guilt that can impede our progress. Make a list of people you feel you may have hurt in the past and how you might have done this. Include the initial reason you acted in this way. Look at each situation a little deeper and see if you can find the real reason you acted in such a way. Perhaps you spread rumors about a coworker because you thought at the time that she was rude and never liked you. Maybe now you can see that you did it because you were jealous of her position in the office.

Once you've written them down, have a "soul conversation" with each person explaining yourself and asking their forgiveness. You can do it right where you are. On a spiritual level, they *will* hear you. Keep it simple and sincere. You might say something like,

"_____, *I know you can hear me because we are together in the great oneness of the universe. I'm sorry for* _____.
I thought I did it because _____.
Looking back, I can see my real motivation was _____
_____. *I ask your forgiveness. Thank you for allowing me to release the guilt attached to this memory. I send you love.*"

Person: _____

_____

What I Did: _____

_____

Initial Reason: _____

_____

Real Reason: _____

NUTRITIONAL RECOMMENDATION

A great way to add good fats to the diet and eliminate starches and sugars is to find healthy alternatives. Switching from commercial peanut butter to almond butter can still satisfy your palate while offering a better-quality fat and more nutrition. You can also switch out white flour pasta for buckwheat pasta, not spinach or tomato pasta. They're still made from wheat flour. Substitute one or two foods today with a healthier version.

DAY 21

THE CORE

Morning Meditation: 15 min.

Exercise/Movement: 30 min.

Gratitude List: 5 things

Evening Meditation: 15 min.

Visualization: 5 min.

YOUR SIDE #4

Honor the Self

On a sheet of paper, write out the entire incident of what happened between you and **the fourth person** you feel has hurt you the most. Be blunt and honest. This is your chance to tell **YOUR** side of the story.

Feel the Experience

When you are finished, imagine the person is sitting in front of you. Read "your story" aloud as if the person where hearing you. Feel free to go "off the page" and speak what's in your heart. Let your feelings flow freely. Don't try to manufacture any specific emotion, but do NOT suppress any that arise. The idea is to FEEL this entire experience. Get your body into it and scream, cry, or punch a pillow if you need to.

When you are finished, destroy the letter in a way that has finality. Don't just throw it away. Burn it, shred it, or some other way that is empowering to you.

That's all you need to do. Take as much time as you need to settle yourself. It's important to reset yourself emotionally by doing something you love, like calling a friend or taking a short walk.

NUTRITIONAL RECOMMENDATION

Develop your taste for spicy foods. Hot spices are very good for digestion, circulation, and cancer prevention. They also work as antimicrobials to keep bad bacteria in the digestive tract at a minimum. Try adding jalapeño, some cayenne pepper, Cajun spices, or mild chili peppers to your diet today. Be careful! A little bit goes a LONG way as they're very hot. You don't need much. Spicy foods should be consumed as condiments in smaller portions, such as in homemade salsa.

DAY 22

THE CORE

Morning Meditation: 15 min.

Exercise/Movement: 30 min.

Gratitude List: 5 things

Evening Meditation: 15 min.

Visualization: 5 min.

FASHION SENSE

Clothes have a very strong ability to make us feel a certain way. They can make us feel powerful, sexy, and beautiful, even if we didn't initially feel that way before we put them on. Make a conscious decision to wear something today that makes you feel powerful, sexy, and beautiful. It might be something new, or an item that's been sitting in the back of your closet for a year because you don't feel worthy enough to wear it. Choose something that accentuates a specific part of your body. A dress hemline that's just an inch or so higher than what you're used to can *really* change how you feel. Lace trim, sheer sleeves, or wearing something that's just a tad more revealing than normal for you can really supercharge how you feel about your body. For men, you may want to wear a sleeveless T-shirt at the gym or try loosening just one extra button on your shirt than you're used to. It's not important that the change even be perceptible to others. The point is that you know the change is there and how it makes YOU feel!

NUTRITIONAL RECOMMENDATION

Protein intake is essential to weight loss and building healthy cells. The easier a protein is to digest, the better these processes work. Choose lighter proteins today, such as eggs and fish. You'll get the benefit of the protein without the stress on your digestive system. You also won't feel as bogged down as if you'd eaten a meal with red meat. Salmon is full of healthy fats, but remember to avoid farm-raised fish of all kinds. Look for labels with "wild caught."

DAY 23

The Core

Morning Meditation: 15 min.

Exercise/Movement: 30 min.

Gratitude List: 5 things

Evening Meditation: 15 min.

Visualization: 5 min.

Rebalance & Release

Re-balancing the Event

After you've honored yourself and fully discharged the emotion of the **Your Side #4** exercise, you can begin to put it into a balanced context. Stand back from the situation and write out the answers to these questions:

1. What belief about myself could this person be revealing to me?

2. Have I been shown this belief from other people in other circumstances?

3. If so, why didn't I react appropriately when I received those messages?

4. This person provided this experience so my life could be changed for the better in what way?

5. What experiences have I had since the incident that verify this improvement?

6. In what way has this person been my teacher?

Once you've re-balanced the event, you can see its perfection in a perfect universe. With this information, complete the forgiveness release below.

Dear _____,

I understand that you came into my life as my partner in learning a powerful lesson. You helped me discover my false belief that _____. Even though

_____ *had to happen for me to understand this, I am grateful for the gifts it has brought me and how it has bettered my life in ways such as* _____

_____. *I understand that this was the best way for me to make this change and that, on the soul level, you chose to help me. I am grateful to you for this gift and know without judgment that your actions came from a place of pure love. I forgive you for any temporary pain I experienced and ask forgiveness for any pain I caused you. Thank you for being my partner in this healing experience. I release it now and we are both free.*

Read the statement out loud and perform the balloon release in a setting that is special to you. Remember to open your arms wide when you release it and watch until it fades out of sight.

Nutritional Recommendation

Breakfast smoothies are a great way to "break" the previous night's fast and give yourself a boost of nutrition and energy instead of a bulky meal. You also won't need the jolt of artificial stimulants like coffee and tea. Instead of your morning meal, make a smoothie today. A simple recipe includes 1 peeled cucumber, ½ green apple, 1 cup of cranberries or blueberries, juice from ½ lemon, ½-inch of ginger root (peeled), ½ an avocado, and 5 ice cubes. Chop and process in a blender until smooth, and enjoy! Have fun with your own combinations.

DAY 24

THE CORE

Morning Meditation: 15 min.

Exercise/Movement: 30 min.

Gratitude List: 5 things

Evening Meditation: 15 min.

Visualization: 5 min..

ME & I

It's time to check in with your inner self. Set two chairs up and conduct the exercise as before. Remember to be open to whatever comes. Affirm those responses when you're back in the "adult" position and provide love and comfort when you speak. Notice how the insights you receive have changed since the beginning of this program.

NUTRITIONAL RECOMMENDATION

We've learned about the transformative power of energy. If energy creates and changes your body, it can change food, too. We're taught to say grace before meals for scientific as well as religious reasons. Loving thoughts and intentions toward your food, such as gratitude, really do change it on an energetic and molecular level. Express sincere gratitude for your food and say grace before each meal today. Be thankful that the food was brought to you, for the money that allowed you to buy it, the farmers who raised it, and the nutrients you will receive from it. If you're eating meat at the meal, thank the living creature that sacrificed its life for your benefit. Say it out loud and be sure your words are heartfelt.

DAY 25

THE CORE

Morning Meditation: 15 min.

Exercise/Movement: 30 min.

Gratitude List: 5 things

Evening Meditation: 15 min.

Visualization: 5 min.

PLAY IT AGAIN

It's time to Play the Part again. Choose another role model whose life or personality you admire. It should be someone who has the kind of life and confidence you want for yourself. Create an imaginary mask of their face that you'll be wearing. Go about your day emulating this person's confidence in your activities. This quite powerful. It gives you permission to act in ways you normally would not because you'll gain a sense of anonymity and safety, allowing you to take some personal or emotional risks.

NUTRITIONAL RECOMMENDATION

Enzymes in our food are essential for our digestion and absorption of nutrients. Cooking foods at high temperatures (over 118-degrees) destroys the enzymes, making them much harder for our bodies to process. Eat an entire meal today of all uncooked or raw foods. This could be a large salad with a smoothie. See how you feel after the meal. When foods are closer to their natural, unprocessed form, they provide more energy (and fewer calories) without the feeling of heaviness. It's not easy to do, but try your best. In time, you'll be able to incorporate more raw foods across all your meals.

DAY 26

THE CORE

Morning Meditation: 15 min.

Exercise/Movement: 30 min.

Gratitude List: 5 things

Evening Meditation: 15 min.

Visualization: 5 min.

KINDNESS OF STRANGERS

This exercise is similar to the role playing you did on the phone earlier. The only difference is that now you can do it in person. Find someone along your daily routine. Maybe you notice an elderly couple on a park bench during your evening walk or there's a seat next to a young couple on the subway. Find a reason to start up a conversation. Perhaps someone is reading a book you're familiar with, or compliment them on something they're wearing. You can always say, "Hello. How are you?" It never fails to get a dialogue going.

Use this opportunity to share details about your "new" life. Let this person know all the wonderful things that are happening. Stay open and be engaging. Because you're having this conversation in person, you'll be able to sustain it a bit longer than a phone chat. As the other person asks questions about your new life, you'll be able to come up with more details that perhaps you hadn't even thought of before. Your conversation is like a string of affirmations that you're putting out into the universe.

NUTRITIONAL RECOMMENDATION

Oftentimes, thyroid conditions can precede or follow a weight gain. The thyroid gland serves a wide range of vital functions, including proper sleep patterns, balancing energy levels, and regulating weight. It requires the trace mineral iodine to function well. Be sure to feed your thyroid today and every day with high-iodine foods. The best choice is sea vegetables (seaweed) like kelp and dulse. You can find these in the Asian section of your grocery store. Some sell shakable versions you can just sprinkle on salads like a spice. If you can't find these, there are plenty of mainstream foods loaded with iodine.

These include cranberries, organic yogurt, organic strawberries, organic goat milk or cheese, and Himalayan brand salt. Never consume large amounts of processed iodized table salt to gain more iodine.

DAY 27

The Core

Morning Meditation: 15 min.

Exercise/Movement: 30 min.

Gratitude List: 5 things

Evening Meditation: 15 min.

Visualization: 5 min.

Dear Diary

Once again, pick up your journal and write the details of a specific day of your "new" life as if it has already happened. Be sure to put a date on it. Choose whatever experience you'd like to have in your new body. Be as descriptive as you can. The more details you provide the more you will feel the experience!

Nutritional Recommendation

Another great switch you can make is to replace your iodized table salt with sea salt. All salt is NOT created equal. Table salt is highly-processed with metals like aluminum to make it pour nicely instead of clumping. Because it's altered from its natural form with iodine added after the fact, our bodies do not recognize it as food. As such, it wreaks havoc on our bodies, particularly blood pressure and the heart. Sea salt is harvested in two ways: either from ancient sea beds within the earth that have long since dried and left their salt behind, or from the current oceans. Because this salt is not processed or combined with additives, our bodies recognize it as food and not an invader. Some great brands include Himalayan, Celtic Sea Salt, and Real Salt. In ancient times, the biological value of salt was so highly valued, it was used as currency. Thus, we still use the phrase today, "He isn't worth his salt."

DAY 28

THE CORE

Morning Meditation: 15 min.

Exercise/Movement: 30 min.

Gratitude List: 5 things

Evening Meditation: 15 min.

Visualization: 5 min.

3 THINGS

We live in a vibrational universe governed by thought and feeling. Manifestation comes when you feel your desire is already here. We want the things we want not so much for the things themselves, but for the way they will make us feel. When we learn to generate those feelings in advance, the things we want manifest quicker. It also takes the pressure off having to "produce" something material. We mind our feelings and the universe creates the material object. That's the universe's arrangement. It takes care of all the details as long as we take care of our emotional state. That's a pretty good deal.

In the space below, write the three biggest ways reaching our ideal weight will make you feel. Perhaps it will make you feel beautiful, sexy, and healthy. In the following space, list things you can do to make yourself experience those feelings *now* through other activities. When you feel beautiful, sexy, and healthy, the universe will send you more things that will help you to continue to feel this way . . . including your ideal weight!

At my ideal weight, I will feel:

1. _____

2. _____

3. _____

I can feel _____ by doing _____

_____.

I can feel _____ by doing _____

_____.

I can feel _____ by doing _____

_____.

Nutritional Recommendation

Eat foods only as they occur in nature. That means avoiding anything that comes from a box, bag or can. You can do this!

DAY 29

THE CORE

Morning Meditation: 15 min.

Exercise/Movement: 30 min.

Gratitude List: 5 things

Evening Meditation: 15 min.

Visualization: 5 min.

ASSET MANAGEMENT

Make a list of all the things you like about yourself. That's it. Just make the list. Be sure to include everything from physical attributes, talents and personality traits to achievements or just something nice you did for someone that you're proud of. This might sound simple, but its effect is enlightening and powerful. It's also very rare that anyone ever does it. You'll be very surprised at how many good things there about you. By the end, you'll be surprised at how much there **really is** to love about you.

NUTRITIONAL RECOMMENDATION

Different enzymes help us digest different kinds of food. Protease helps us digest protein, while lipase helps us digest fat, and so on. Certain foods require specific enzymes and digestive processes, while others need something else. Eating certain foods together or those with longs lists of ingredients can send confusing messages to our body as to what kind of digestive process it needs to prepare for. The process and enzymes needed for digesting meat are different than those needed for fruit. Mixing foods up can create digestive havoc on our bodies. The general rule is to do your best not to eat protein and starches at the same time. That means no meat with bread, pasta, or potatoes. Eating meat with vegetables is a beneficial combination. Fruit should always be eaten by itself or in advance of a meal, as it digests very quickly. Apply these two simple rules to your meals today and see how healthier food combinations affect you.

DAY 30

THE CORE

Morning Meditation: 15 min.

Exercise/Movement: 30 min.

Gratitude List: 5 things

Evening Meditation: 15 min.

Visualization: 5 min.

PRESS CONFERENCE

Imagine *you* are a bestselling author who has just written a wildly successful book on weight loss (or any goal you'd like to achieve). You're at a book signing and press conference, facing 30 or 40 reporters. Light bulbs are flashing as they shout out questions to you. Everyone wants to know how you did it and what your life is like in your new slim physique.

Think about the kinds of questions you might be asked. Write them down and before the exercise, record them into a digital recorder or your cell phone. Try to ask questions that focus on how you FEEL in your new body and life, what your future plans are, how you lost the weight, and what advice you'd give to others.

Once you have 10-12 really good questions, close your eyes and imagine yourself at the press conference. Hear the voices. See the cameras flash. Feel your hand signing a few books. With your eyes still closed, hit the play button on your recorder. Once the first question is asked, pause the recorder and take as long as you like to answer, in as much detail as possible. Press the play button again when you're ready for the second question. Keep your eyes closed and really visualize each individual reporter who is asking the question.

Get into this. Make it fun and feel the sense of accomplishment and pride at having achieved your weight loss, and the gratitude of being able to help others through your experience. Once again, you're putting these words out into the universe in a fun but very real way.

Nutritional Recommendation

Eating more vegetables can be a challenge, especially if you're trying to consume them in their raw form. That's a lot of chewing! The best way to consume vegetables is through juicing. If you have a juicer, mix leafy greens like Swiss chard, collard green, and kale with some carrot and half a green apple. You can make any combination you like. Juicing allows your body to take up the minerals and chlorophyll from the vegetables almost immediately. You can consume ten times more vegetables this way and you'll be amazed at what it does for your skin. If you don't have a juicer, you can use a blender. Strain the liquid out of the mix with some cheesecloth and throw the pulp away. Increase your vegetable volume with juicing today. I don't recommend store juices because of the added sugars. You'll want to invest in a home juicer for its many health benefits. Avoid juicing fruits, as the concentrated sugar without its pulp will enter your bloodstream too quickly.

DAY 31

THE CORE

Morning Meditation: 15 min.

Exercise/Movement: 30 min.

Gratitude List: 5 things

Evening Meditation: 15 min.

Visualization: 5 min.

FACE OFF / SLIM DOWN

Where we place our attention is very important in manifesting things in our lives. Much of our attention includes what we choose to focus on visually. Get some magazines and find pictures of the kind of body you'd like to have. Find images of people in various forms of dress: formalwear, swimsuits, business attire, and street clothes. Cut out these images and paste them onto a piece of poster board or in a scrapbook. Lastly, make photocopies of a photograph of your face that you like. Cut out just your face and paste it over top of the models' faces in the pictures. Look at this collage regularly as a way to help you visualize and see yourself at your goal weight.

If you or someone you know has skill using graphic design software such as Photoshop, there's an even better way to do this exercise. Find a recent full-length picture of you that you like. Using the software, alter the image to slim your figure to the size that you desire. Make any other changes you like. Because this image is *completely* you and not a cut-and-paste, your subconscious can accept it more readily.

NUTRITIONAL RECOMMENDATION

Fiber is important for many health reasons, including weight loss. You should be getting enough fiber through your increased vegetable intake. If it's still a problem or you're having trouble with regularity, you'll need to add a bit more. Unhealthy processed foods have very little fiber, causing them to stagnate in our organs of elimination, creating toxicity that can make us sick. Choose natural fibers, such as ground flaxseed or chia seed mixes. These can be sprinkled into foods in small amounts or added to your morning smoothie.

DAY 32

THE CORE

Morning Meditation: 15 min.

Exercise/Movement: 30 min.

Gratitude List: 5 things

Evening Meditation: 15 min.

Visualization: 5 min.

ME & I

It's time to check in with your inner self. Set two chairs up and conduct the exercise as before. Remember to be open to whatever comes. Affirm those responses when you're back in the "adult" position and provide love and comfort when you speak. Notice how the insights you receive have changed since the beginning of this exercise.

NUTRITIONAL RECOMMENDATION

A great way to keep good fats in proportion is to order them on the side during a meal. Stick your fork into the oil before it goes into the salad. The oil that clings to the fork tines will be more than enough flavor to satisfy you without pouring too much over the entire salad. This trick can be used with most condiments, like ketchup, which hides a lot of sugar and calories. Try this during your meals today and stay open to the realization of quality of flavor over quantity of the serving.

DAY 33

THE CORE

Morning Meditation: 15 min.

Exercise/Movement: 30 min.

Gratitude List: 5 things

Evening Meditation: 15 min.

Visualization: 5 min.

PLAYING THE ODDS

With universal laws stacked so high in your favor, the odds are tremendous that you will achieve whatever you want in life as long as you remain in the flow of good-feeling vibrations. In the space below, list as many reasons as you can for why you will succeed in reaching your ideal weight. Some reasons might include that people all over the world lose weight and maintain the loss every single day. The universe says whatever you sow you will reap, and you are putting all the right messages out into the world. You have a loving and supportive family. List as many as you can and you'll see that all the odds really are on your side.

_____

_____

_____

_____

_____

_____

_____

_____

_____

_____

_____

Nutritional Recommendation

Believe it or not, when we sniff certain foods, our hunger mechanism shuts off because our brain thinks we're actually eating them. There's real science behind this and it seems to work best with a banana, an apple, or peppermint. Give this a try tonight if the after-8:00 p.m. munchies hit.

DAY 34

THE CORE

Morning Meditation: 15 min.

Exercise/Movement: 30 min.

Gratitude List: 5 things

Evening Meditation: 15 min.

Visualization: 5 min.

THE YES FACTOR

So much of bringing what we want into our lives depends on staying in a good emotional place. Too often, we let the little things drag us onto a negative emotional track, and then the whole day is ruined. Today, you're going to say YES to everything that comes along. No resistance. If a restaurant is out of your favorite dish, say, "YES. Now I can try something new for a change." If a friend cancels your dinner date say, "YES. Now I can stay home and catch up on my reading." If you get a big project dumped on you at work, say, "YES. Now I know I'm still valuable to the company." If you get laid off say, "YES. Now I can find a job that's more fulfilling to me." It can be hard to always say YES, but the Law of Attraction is AFFIRMATIVE. The more you turn negatives situations into YES moments, the more power you'll have to bring good things into your life. How can you say YES to your weight loss process?

NUTRITIONAL RECOMMENDATION

By avoiding processed sugar and most starches, your tastes will change. This is inevitable, but you have to stay away from these items for about 30 days before the change is apparent. Test yourself today and do not eat anything containing sugar, processed or natural. This will be a challenge, but you'll know right away from the strength of the cravings or withdrawal symptoms (like headache) that you experience how close you are to not being a slave to sugar anymore.

DAY 35

THE CORE

Morning Meditation: 15 min.

Exercise/Movement: 30 min.

Gratitude List: 5 things

Evening Meditation: 15 min.

Visualization: 5 min.

For the Love of It

The Law of Attraction is love in action. See how many times today you can focus on things you love. It could be the weather, someone's dress, the décor in your office, a specific kind of car on the street, or anything else meaningful to you. Be on the lookout. Notice all the little things there are to love in a day. Keep yourself in a loving mode. In fact, say, "I LOVE that," out loud, even if you're alone. It will heighten your awareness of what it means to really stay in a loving state all day long.

NUTRITIONAL RECOMMENDATION

You've heard it before, but it bears repeating. Water is invaluable to your health and weight loss efforts. Your body is roughly 70% water. To search for life on other planets, scientists look for one thing: water. It's elemental to life. Our very existence depends on it. Increasing your water intake will accelerate your weight loss and improve your health exponentially. How much is enough? The general rule is to multiply your weight by .65. This means a 200-lb. man should consume 130-oz or 1.02 gallons of water daily. Other liquids don't count. This is pure water. See if you can consume the proper amount for weight today.

DAY 36

THE CORE

Morning Meditation: 15 min.

Exercise/Movement: 30 min.

Gratitude List: 5 things

Evening Meditation: 15 min.

Visualization: 5 min.

THANK YOU UNIVERSE

This exercise is designed to help you feel deep gratitude, as well as the idea that your ideal weight has already arrived. In the space below, write a thank-you note to the universe. Tell the universe how grateful you are to have your ideal weight, because now you can play with your kids, walk up stairs without being winded, sit comfortably in a cinema or on an airplane, or you can take the trips now that you've always wanted to. There are thousands of things you can be thankful for about your new life. Write a very sincere note below, as if it's already happened.

Dear Universe,

I am grateful that:

_____

_____

_____

_____

_____

_____

_____

_____

_____

Nutritional Recommendation

I believe in the benefit of whole, unprocessed dairy products—that is, if you can find them today. Nearly all commercial dairy products are pasteurized, homogenized, filled with animal growth hormones, and mixed with Vitamin D additives that were previously destroyed during the processing phases. After this transformation, little is left in the milk except the sugar . . . and there's a lot of sugar in milk. Check the labels. Instead of milk, I suggest drinking low-sugar kefir or learning how to make it yourself. It's very simple. You can find great information on culturesforhealth.com. An easier substitution for commercial milk is to switch to almond milk. You can find it in most grocery stores. Be sure to choose a brand with little or no sugar. The consistency is closer to skim milk. You can add a touch of honey, if it suits you. Add it to a morning smoothie and see how you like it.

DAY 37

THE CORE

Morning Meditation: 15 min.

Exercise/Movement: 30 min.

Gratitude List: 5 things

Evening Meditation: 15 min.

Visualization: 5 min.

PRIVATE DANCER

Our bodies are very powerful tools to our psyches. Because our bodies and minds are connected, what happens in one must be echoed in the other. Tension in our minds transfers to our shoulders, jaw, neck, and so on. Put on one of your favorite pieces of music in a place where you're uninhibited and won't be disturbed. Move in any way the music dictates to you. Don't feel like you need to do a specific dance of any kind. That's too logical, too left-brained. Allow the music to flow through you and express itself in any way it chooses to. Music is vibration and its effect on us is powerful. This exercise allows you to get "out of your head" and into your body. This can be a very freeing and enjoyable experience. Do it for as long as you desire, and then sit quietly and notice the sensations in your body. What do you feel? What is it telling you?

NUTRITIONAL RECOMMENDATION

Artificial sweeteners are as bad as sugar. They actually make you gain weight. How? The fake sweet taste tells the brain that sugar is on the way. When no calories from sugar appear in your bloodstream, the brain gets confused and never gives you the chemical signal that it's satisfied. So, the craving never shuts off as it drives you to consume more of the real thing: sugar. This isn't even taking into consideration the chemicals these substances are made from. Avoid all foods with artificial sweeteners. If you have a sugar craving, eat an apple instead!

DAY 38

THE CORE

Morning Meditation: 15 min.

Exercise/Movement: 30 min.

Gratitude List: 5 things

Evening Meditation: 15 min.

Visualization: 5 min.

TO DO LIST

Most people have a list of things they'd like to do in their lives, but feel they can't until "X" happens. The problem with this approach is that it's a life projected into the future, not a NOW-centered way of living. So, "X" never arrives because the future will always be . . . in the future. It's not NOW.

Make a list of all the things you really want to do *after* you've reached your goal weight. If I could write a prescription that was perfectly tailored to your individual healing, it would be *this list*. This is your prescription for healing. These are the things you're telling your body you will do once you are thin. Start doing these things NOW. Start sending the message to your body that you've already lost the weight and it will cooperate with you! This is your To Do List for however long it takes to complete all the activities, big and small alike. Do just one of them today.

When I reach my goal weight I will:

_____

_____

_____

_____

_____

_____

_____

Nutritional Recommendation

When you eat in, you almost always eat healthier. There is no restaurant that could ever make anything as healthy as you could when you control the ingredients and preparation. Today, prepare all your meals at home—no eating out. It may help to prepare meals the night before, particularly for your lunch at work. Preparing food regularly is also a great way to re-establish a cooperative and positive relationship with food. Cooking and providing sustenance for someone, particularly our families is a very nurturing process. You can learn to nurture yourself through the same process, too.

DAY 39

THE CORE

Morning Meditation: 15 min.

Exercise/Movement: 30 min.

Gratitude List: 5 things

Evening Meditation: 15 min.

Visualization: 5 min.

BODY CONTACT

Just as you did on Day 14, lie in a comfortable place where you will not be disturbed. Keep the lights dimmed and begin at the top of your head and work all the way to the tips of your toes. Talk to each part of your body in a loving, grateful way. Be appreciative of all it does for you on a daily basis that you're not even aware of. Be sure your touch is comforting, like that of a parent. Pay attention to your comfort levels during this exercise. How have they changed in the past weeks? How has your relationship with your body changed in this moment?

NUTRITIONAL RECOMMENDATION

If you asked me what the single most important dietary change you could make that would impact your health and weight is, I would say this. Our health and weight will return to normal faster based more on what we *don't* eat rather than what we do eat. The Big Bad 4 are sugar, artificial sweeteners, white flour and its products, and margarine. We've spoken of the previous three. Margarine is loaded with polyunsaturated fat, trans fats, and hydrogenated vegetable oil. Do you want to know how unfit for human consumption it is? Leave a stick out on your kitchen counter. What happens months later? Nothing. It will remain absolutely unchanged. Mold will not grow on it. That's how nutritionally void it is. It can't even support the life of a single-celled organism. It's just not food. Always use butter. You'll be further in your weight loss goals if you do nothing else but avoid these four dangerous items.

DAY 40

THE CORE

Morning Meditation: 15 min.

Exercise/Movement: 30 min.

Gratitude List: 5 things

Evening Meditation: 15 min.

Visualization: 5 min.

A NEW YOU

Get one more helium-filled balloon. This one is for you. Make sure it's a color or design that is special to you. You'll also want to get a single flower. The iris is the symbol of rebirth and renewal. Queen Anne's lace (which can be found in almost any backyard) is the symbol of grace. The rose of course, symbolizes love. Any flower will do as long as it carries significance for you.

Think about all you've been through the last 40 days. Reflect on your experiences, revealed emotions, and risks taken. Fill yourself up with the gratitude of this journey. On a note card, write the words, "Thank you. I am free." Tie it to the balloon's ribbon. Hold it to your heart. Then, release it. Stay in this moment as long as you need. Place the flower in a vase as your personal symbol of renewal. It will be the constant reminder throughout the coming days that you are significantly changed within . . . and without.

NUTRITIONAL RECOMMENDATION

Remember that deprivation only leads to overindulgence later on. If you give yourself something to work toward, a "splurge meal" on Saturday night, you'll find it much easier to stick to better food choices throughout the week. No matter how much of a guilty pleasure your weekend meal may be, there's no way to negate six days of good eating with one "bad" dinner. Just be sure to eat it with joy and no guilt. That way, you'll be able to return to your healthy habits with a sense of satisfaction and accomplishment.

ABOUT THE HEALING INSTITUTE OF BEINGS (HIB)

The Healing Institute of Beings (HIB) is a nonprofit, 501c3 organization that combines integrative medicine with ancient holistic healing traditions to create a comprehensive healing strategy that transforms the soul, while rebuilding the body. The medical component includes the latest advances in Western evidence-based medicine, as well as integrative, anthroposophical, osteopathic, homeopathic and integrative bio-regulatory medicine (iBm). Complementing the medical component is a wide range of time-tested Eastern healing modalities such as Ayurveda, acupuncture, detoxification and many others.

Because we cannot solve a problem from the same level of consciousness that created it, HIB incorporates a separate healing protocol for the mind and soul. Spiritual sharing is encouraged, and direction is provided in ways to bring positive healing energy back into life. We all want answers, and guidance is provided to find purpose and meaning, especially during difficult times. This component also provides guided meditation, sound resonance with directed intention and energy healing based on pre-set goals. These interventions elevate the way one thinks, feels and processes life events, which always affect physical health.

The core of HIB's mission is to bring awareness of true body/mind/soul healing to the world in a way that's accessible and enlightening. To do this, we conduct healing conferences all across the U.S. and Canada, to create a bridge between spiritual education and healing dynamics. It's time for a paradigm shift in the way we think of health, and we're doing our best to "be" the change we want to see in the world.

In addition, HIB is involved in a number of outreach programs and partnering with other nonprofit organizations to promote education, increase access to nutritious food and other notable causes. Some of these include:

Campus Intervention: Reaching out to college students on campus where a crime or crisis occurred.

LoveButton.org: Launched a fun and interactive website to encourage Random Acts of Love.

Prison Outreach: Sponsoring theater programs that bring creativity and inspiration to inmates.

Endowments: Establishing endowments to ensure future medical students receive true holistic healing education.

Educating Children: Partnering with programs like The Virginia Avenue Project to help children graduate and get into college.

Feeding Children: Partnering with Nourish the Children to bring healthy meals to those in need around the world.

HIB was co-founded by **Dr. Habib Sadeghi** and **Sri Madhuji**. Dr. Sadeghi is the co-founder of Be Hive of Healing, an integrative medical center in Los Angeles. Sri Maduji studied as a monk under Sri Bhagavan for twelve years before leaving the order to provide spiritual healing services around the world. You can reach HIB at: www.healingbeings.org.

ENDNOTES

1. Andreyeva T, Puhl RM, Brownell KD. Changes in perceived weight discrimination among Americans: 1995–1996 through 2004–2006. Obesity (Silver Spring) 2008;16: 1129–1134.

2. Roehling MV, Roehling PV, Pichler S. The relationship between body weight and perceived weight-related employment discrimination: the role of sex and race. J Vocat Behav 2007;71:300–318.

3. Foster GD, Wadden TA, Makris AP, et al. Primary care physicians' attitudes about obesity and its treatment. Obes Res 2003;11: 1168–1177.

4. Brown I. Nurses' attitudes towards adult patients who are obese: literature review. J Adv Nurs 2006;53:221–232.

5. McCraty, R. The energetic heart: : bioelectromagnetic communication within and between people. Clinical Applications of Bioelectromagnetic Medicine 2004; 541-562.

6. Greene, Brian. *The Elegant Universe: Superstrings, Hidden Dimensions and the Quest for the Ultimate Theory.* 1st. New York: Random House, 2003. 124-125. Print.

7. Buhlman, William. *Adventures Beyond the Body.* 1st. San Francisco: HarperCollins, 1996. 96. Print.

8. Bergmann, O., Bhardwaj, R. D., Bernard, S., Zdunek, S., Barnabe-Heider, F., Walsh, S., Zupicich, J., Alkass, K., Buchholz, B. A., Druid, H., et al. (2009). *Evidence for cardiomyocyte renewal in humans. Science* 324, 98-102.

9. Chopra, Ph.D., Deepak. "Living Beyond Miracles." Living Beyond Miracles with Deepak Chopra & Wayne Dyer. Church of Today. Warren, MI. 1992. Lecture.

10. Bradshaw, John. *Family Secrets: The Path to Self-Acceptance and Reunion.* First edition. Bantam Doubleday Dell Publishing Group, 1995. Print.

11. Winter, Deena. "Financial Planners: Winning the lottery isn't always a dream. " *Lincoln Journal Star* 26 February 2006, Print.

12. Bitzer, Robert. The collected essays of Robert Bitzer. Second. Marina del Rey, CA: Devorss & Co, 1990. 136-137. Print.

13. Kuhn Truman, Karol. *Feelings Buried Alive Never Die.* First. Las Vegas: Olympus Distributing, 1991. Print.

14. Lewis, M. Paul. "Languages of the World." *Ethnologue* 2009: n. pag. Web. 4 Mar 2011. <http://citationmachine.net/ index2hp?reqstyleid=1&mode=form&reqsrcid=MLAMagazine Online&more=yes&nameCnt=1>.

15. M., Sheila, and Katharine Fairlie. *Anatomy and physiology for nurses.* 9th. London: Bailliere Tindall: Harcourt College Pub, 1979. Print.

16. Emoto, Masaru. *The hidden messages in water.* Hillsboro, Oregon: Beyond Words Publishing Co, 2004. Print.

17. Allen, James. *As A Man Thinketh.* 2007. New York: Barnes & Nobel, Inc., 2007. 13. Print.

18. Schucman, Helen. *A Course in Miracles.* 3rd. Mill Valley, CA: Foundation for Inner Peace, 2007, Print.

19. Goddard, Neville. *Feeling IS the Secret.* 5th. United States: 1944. Print.

20. Eliot, Marc. *Cary Grant: A Biography.* New York: Three Rivers Press, 2004. Print.

21. Schwarz, Benjamin. "Becoming Cary Grant." *The Atlantic.* January/ February 2007: n. pag. Web. 13 Mar 2011. <http://www.theatlantic.com/ magazine/archive/2007/01/becoming-cary-grant/5548.>

22. Wattles, Wallace D. *The Science of Getting Rich: Attracting Financial Success Through Creative Thought.* Rochester, VT: Destiny Book, 1976. Print.

23. Feinberg, Cara. "The Mindfulness Chronicles: On The Psychology of Possibility." *Harvard Magazine* September-October 2010: 42-46. Web. 13 Mar 2011. <http://harvardmag.com/pdf/2010/09-pdfs/0910-42.pdf>.

24. Byrne, Rhonda. *The Secret.* First. Hillsboro, Oregon: Beyond Words Publishing, 2006. 81. Print.

25. A. Pascual-Leone, D. Nguyet, L.G. Cohen, J.P. Brasil-Neto, A.

Cammarota, and M. Hallet, "Modulation of muscle responses evoked by transcranial magnetic stimulation during the acquisition of new fine motor skills," *Journal of Neurophysiology,* 1995, 74(3), 1037-45.

26. V.K. Ranganathan, V. Siemionow, J.Z. Liu, V. Sahgal, and G.H. Yue, "From mental power to muscle power—gaining strength by using the mind," *Neuropsychologia,* 2004, 42(7), 944-56.

27. C.A. Porro, P. Facchin, S. Fusi, G, Dri, and L. Fadiga, "Enhancement of force after action observation: behavioral and neurophysiological studies," *Neuropsychologia,* 2007, 45(13), 3114-21.

28. A. Guillot, F. Lebon, D. Rouffet, S. Champely, J. Doyon, and C. Collet, "Muscular responses during motor imagery as a function of muscle contraction types," *International Journal of Psychophysiology,* 2007, 66(1), 18-27.

29. D. Ertelt, S. Small, A. Solodkin, C. Dettmers, A. McNamara, F. Binkofski, and G. Buccino, "Action observation has a positive impact on rehabilitation of motor deficits after stroke," *Neuroimage,* 2007, 36, Supplement 2, T164-73.

30. Marketdata Enterprises, Inc., *MarketResearch.com.* Marketdata Enterprises, Inc., April 1, 2010. Web. 21 Mar 2011. <http://www.marketresearch.com/map/prod/2641578.html>.

31. "About the Industry." *International Health, Racquet and Sportsclub Association.* IHRSA, January 2010. Web. 21 Mar 2011. <http://www.ihrsa.org/about-the-industry/>.

32. *www.Surgery.org.* American Society for Aesthetic Plastic Surgery, 2009. Web. 21 Mar 2011. <http://www.surgery.org/sites/default/files/2009stats.pdf>.

33. "Beauty at Any Cost: The Consequences of America's Beauty Obsession on Women & Girls." *www.ywca.org.* YWCA, August 2008. Web. 21 Mar 2011. <http://www.ywca.org/atf/cf/%7B3B450FA5-108B-4D2E-B3D0-C31487243E6A%7D/Beauty%20at%20Any%20Cost.pdf>.

34. Karras, Tula. "Disordered Eating: The disorder next door." *SELF magazine* 2008: n. pag. Web. 21 Mar 2011. <http://www.self.com/

fooddiet/2008/04/eating-disorder-risk>.

35. Winterman, Denise. "What would a real life Barbie look like?" *BBC News Magazine* March 6, 2009: n. pag. Web. 21 Mar 2011. <http://news.bbc.co.uk/2/hi/uk_news/magazine/7920962.stm>.

36. Fouts, G., & Burggraf, K. (1999). Television situation comedies: Female body images and verbal reinforcements. *Sex Roles, 40*(5/6), 473-481.

37. Hudson, James I. M.D., Sc.D., et al. The Prevalence and Correlates of Eating Disorders in the National Comorbidity Survey Replication. *Biological Psychiatry*. February 2007.

38. Bryner, Jeanna. "Steamy magazines make men feel as bad as women." *LiveScience* November 7, 2008: n. pag. Web. 22 Mar 2011. <http://www.livescience.com/3029-steamy-magazines-men-feel-bad-women.html>.

39. Phillips, Olivardia, Harrison, Katharine, Roberto. *The Adonis Complex: How to identify, treat and prevent body obsession in men and boys*. First. New York: Touchstone Books, 2002. Print.

40. Cromie, William J. "Drugs muscle their way into men's fitness." *Harvard Gazette* June 15, 2000, Print.

41. Pope, H. G., Olivardia, R., Gruber, A., & Borowiecki, J. (1999). Evolving ideals of male body image as seen through action toys. International Journal of Eating Disorders, 26(1), 65-72.

42. Shapiro Barash, Susan. *Tripping the Prom Queen: The Truth about Women and Rivalry*. First. New York: St. Martin's Press, 2006. Print.

43. "After Gastric Bypass Surgery, Women Battle Alcoholism." *Good Morning America*. ABC News Network: WABC7, Los Angeles, July 19, 2006. Web. 24 Mar 2011. <http://abcnews.go.com/GMA/story?id=2210783&page=1>.

44. Baranski Sons, Kelly. "Addiction Transfer: Bypass to Alcoholism." *Associated Content* July 2, 2007: n. pag. Web. 24 Mar 2011. <http://www.associatedcontent.com/article/293817/addiction_transfer_bypass_to_alcoholism.html?cat=5>.

45. White, Tracie. "Bariatric surgery can make more people sensitive to alcohol, Stanford surgeon finds." *Stanford School of Medicine*. Stanford University, June 14, 2007. Web. 24 Mar 2011. <http://med.stanford.edu/news_releases/2007/june/bariatric.html>.

46. Woodard, Downey, Hernandez-Boussard, Morton, Gavitt A, John, Tina, John M. "Impaired Alcohol Metabolism after Gastric Bypass Surgery: A Case-Crossover Trial." *Journal of the American College of Surgeons*. 212.2 (2010): 209-214. Print.

47. Squires, Sally. "Optimal Weight Threshold Lowered." *Washington Post* June 4, 1998: A01. Print.

48. Wechsler, Pat. "Teen Girls' Fat Surgery May Raise Birth Defect, Study Says." *Bloomberg News* Oct. 3, 2010: n. pag. Web. 26 Mar 2011. <http://www.bloomberg.com/news/2010-10-03/teen-girls-fat-surgery-may-raise-birth-defect-risk-study-says.html>.

49. Richwine, Lisa. "FDA Considers Lap Band Surgery for Less Obese." *MSNBC.com* Dec. 2, 2010: n. pag. Web. 26 Mar 2011. <http://www.msnbc.msn.com/id/40476329/ns/health-diet_and_nutrition/>.

50. Pollack, Andrew. "Obesity Surgery May Become Option for Many More." *New York Times* Dec. 1 2010, Business DayPrint.

51. Richwine, Lisa. "FDA Considers Lap Band Surgery for Less Obese." *MSNBC.com* Dec. 2, 2010: n. pag. Web. 26 Mar 2011. <http://www.msnbc.msn.com/id/40476329/ns/health-diet_and_nutrition/>.

52. Wechsler, Pat. "Obesity Lap Bands Cause More Complications Than Weight Loss, Study Finds." *Bloomberg News* March 21, 2011: n. pag. Web. 26 Mar 2011. <http://www.bloomberg.com/news/2011-03-21/obesity-lap-bands-may-cause-more-complications-than-weight-loss.html>.

53. Tasi, Inge, Randall, Burd, Wilson S., Thomas H., Randall S. "Bariatric Surgery in Adolescents: Recent national trends in use and in-hospital outcomes." *Archives of Pediatrics and Adolescent Medicine* 161.3 (2007): 217-221.

54. Pappas, Stephanie. "Obese Teens Prefer Gastric Bands Over Gastric Bypass." *LiveScience* Sept. 20, 2010: n. pag. Web. 28 Mar 2011. <http://

www.livescience.com/8615-obese-teens-prefer-gastric-bands-gastric-bypass.html>.

55. Wechsler, Pat. "Teen Girls' Fat Surgery May Raise Birth Defect, Study Says." *Bloomberg News* Oct. 3, 2010: n. pag. Web. 26 Mar 2011. <http://www.bloomberg.com/news/2010-10-03/teen-girls-fat-surgery-may-raise-birth-defect-risk-study-says.html>.

56. Biel, Laura. "Surgery for Obese Children?" *New York Times* Feb. 15, 2010: n. pag. Web. 28 Mar 2011. <http://www.nytimes.com/2010/02/16/health/16teen.html?pagewanted=1&_r=2>.

57. Ippisch, Jenkins, Inge, Kimball, Holly M., Todd M., Thomas H., Thomas R. "Do Acute Improvements in LV Mass and Diastolic Function Following Adolescent Bariatric Surgery Persist at Two Years Post-Op?" *Circulation: American Heart Association Journals.* S474. (2009): 120. Print.

58. O'Brien, Paul, *et al.* "Laparoscopic Adjustable Gastric Banding in Severely Obese Adolescents." *Journal of the American Medical Association* 303.6 (2010): 519-526. Web. 28 Mar 2011. <http://jama.ama-assn.org/content/303/6/519.full?home>.

59. "Overweight People Live Longer." *West Australian: Yahoo News* June 18, 2009: n. pag. Web. 28 Mar 2011. <http://au.news.yahoo.com/thewest/lifestyle/a/-/health/5805835/overweight-people-live-longer-study/>.

60. Mate, Dr. Gabor. *Zeitgeist: Moving Forward* Interview by Peter Joseph. Gentle Machine Productions, March 1, 2011. Genetics. Film. 2 Apr 2011.

61. *The Biology of Perception: The Psychology of Change, Piecing It All Together.* Perf. Lipton, Ph.D., Bruce. Spirit 2000, Inc.: 2001, DVD.

62. Chopra, Ph.D., Deepak. "Living Beyond Miracles." Living Beyond Miracles with Deepak Chopra & Wayne Dyer. Church of Today. Warren, MI. 1992. Lecture.

63. Heijmans, Bastiaan, T. "Persistent epigenetic differences associated with prenatal exposure to famine in humans." *Proceedings of the National Academy of Science of the United States of America* 105.44 (2008): 17046-17049. Web. 2 Apr 2011. <http://www.pnas.org/content/105/44/17046.long>.

64. Birky CW Jr. Uniparental inheritance of mitochondrial and chloroplast genes: mechanisms and evolution. *Proc Natl Acad Sci* U S A 1995;92: 11331-8.

65. Saplosky, Dr. Robert, professor of neurological sciences, Stanford University. *Zeitgeist: Moving Forward.* Interview by Peter Joseph. Gentle Machine Productions, March 1, 2011. Genetics. Film. 2 Apr 2011.

66. Siegel, Bernie S., M.D. *Love, Medicine & Miracles: Lessons learned about self-healing from a surgeon's experience with exceptional patients.* First. New York: HarperCollins Publishing, 1988. Print.

67. Streib, Lauren. "World's Fattest Countries." *Forbes Magazine* Feb. 8, 2007: n. pag. Web. 7 Apr 2011. <http://www.forbes.com/2007/02/07/worlds-fattest-countries-forbeslife-cx_ls_0208worldfat.html>.

68. David, Marc. *Nourishing Wisdom: A Mind-Body Approach to Nutrition and Well-being.* First. New York, New York: Crown Publishing Group, 1994. Print.

69. Buettner, Dan. *The Blue Zones: Lessons for living longer from the people who have lived the longest.* First. Washington D.C.: National Geographic Society, 2008. Print.

70. Cousins, Norman. *Anatomy of an Illness.* 20th. New York: W.W. Norton & Company, 2005. Print.

71. Ophir, Nass, Wagner, Eyal, Clifford, Anthony D. "Cognitive Control in Media Multitaskers." *Proceedings of the National Academy of Science of the United States of America* Aug.24 (2009): 1-5. Web. 12 Apr 2011. <http://www.pnas.org/content/early/2009/08/21/0903620106.abstract>.

72. Foerde, Knowlton, Poldrack, Karin, Barbara A., Russell J. "Modulation of competing memory systems by distraction." *Proceedings of the National Academy of Sciences of the United States of America* 103.31 (2006): 11778-11783. Web. 12 Apr 2011. <http://www.pnas.org/content/103/31/11778.full>.

73. Connelly, Marjorie. "More Americans Sense a Downside to an Always Plugged-In Existence." *New York Times* June 6, 2010, Print.

74. Richtel, Matt. "Your Brain on Computers: Outdoors and Out of Reach, Studying the Brain." *New York Times* August 15, 2010, Print.

75. Andersen, U.S. *Three Magic Words.* Chatsworth, CA: Wilshire Book Company, 1954. 122. Print.

76. McCraty, Ph.D., Rollin, Atkinson, Mike, Tomasion, B.A., Dana, Tiller, William. "The Electricity of Touch: Detection and Measurement of Cardiac Energy Exchange between People." *Lawrence Erlbaum Associates, Publishers,* (1998): 359-379. Web. 31 May 2011. <http://www. heartmath.org/research/research-publications/electricity-of-touch-page-3.html>.

77. G. Rein, R, McCraty. Local and non-local effects of coherent heart frequencies on conformational changes of DNA. Proc. Joint USPA/ IAPR Conference, Milwaukee, WI 1993. http://appreciativeinquiry.case. edu/uploads/HeartMath%20article

ABOUT THE AUTHOR

Dr. Habib Sadeghi, DO, is the cofounder of Be Hive of Healing, an integrative health center based in Los Angeles. He is a highly respected physician and researcher in the fields of integrative, osteopathic, anthroposophical, environmental, family, and German new medicine, as well as homeopathy and clinical pharmacology. He has served as an attending physician and clinical facilitator at UCLA–Santa Monica Medical Center, as well as a clinical instructor of family medicine at Western University of Health Sciences. He is a member of the Physician's Association for Anthroposophic Medicine and the International Post-Graduate Medical Training for Anthroposophic Medicine. An active member of the Price-Pottenger Nutrition Foundation and the American Holistic Medical Association, he is regularly sought after as an expert in the fields of nutritional therapy, dietary supplementation, and detoxification for chronic conditions such as heart disease, cancer, and autoimmune diseases at venues around the world.

Having recovered from cancer decades ago through his unique combination of integrative medical protocols, his services are in great demand. His patients come from as far as Columbia, Mexico, Germany, Thailand, France, Canada, Israel, and the United Kingdom, seeking his specialized combination of integrative therapies.

Dr. Sadeghi serves as an on-air health expert for Fox News and *Geraldo at Large*. He is coauthor of the book *The Light*, along with renowned spiritual teachers Don Miguel Ruiz (*The Four Agreements*), Terry Tillman (*Writings on the Wall*), Barbara Marx Hubbard (*Emergence: Shift from Ego to Essence*), John-Roger (*Living the Spiritual Principles of Health and Wellbeing*) and Marci Shimoff (coauthor of the Chicken Soup for the Soul series and *Love for No Reason*). He was also one of the first two osteopathic physicians ever to be included as a medical expert in the nationally televised cancer research fundraising telethon Stand Up to Cancer (SU2C), executive produced by Gwyneth Paltrow. He is the publisher of Be Hive of Healing Medical Corporation's monthly newsletter and the spiritual health magazine *MegaZen*.

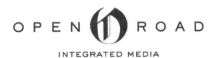

OPEN ROAD

INTEGRATED MEDIA

Open Road Integrated Media is a digital publisher and multimedia content company. Open Road creates connections between authors and their audiences by marketing its ebooks through a new proprietary online platform, which uses premium video content and social media.

WITHIN

CPSIA information can be obtained
at www.ICGtesting.com
Printed in the USA
BVOW08s1139100118
504960BV00004B/353/P